GENERATION CARE

THE NEW CULTURE OF CAREGIVING

GENERATION CARE

JENNIFER N. LEVIN

balance

New York Boston

Copyright © 2025 by Jennifer N. Levin
Cover design by Terri Sirma
Cover copyright © 2025 by Hachette Book Group, Inc.

Hachette Book Group supports the right to free expression and the value of copyright. The purpose of copyright is to encourage writers and artists to produce the creative works that enrich our culture.

The scanning, uploading, and distribution of this book without permission is a theft of the author's intellectual property. If you would like permission to use material from the book (other than for review purposes), please contact Permissions@hbgusa.com. Thank you for your support of the author's rights.

Balance
Hachette Book Group
1290 Avenue of the Americas
New York, NY 10104
GCP-Balance.com
@GCPBalance

First Edition: April 2025

Balance is an imprint of Grand Central Publishing. The Balance name and logo are registered trademarks of Hachette Book Group, Inc.

The publisher is not responsible for websites (or their content) that are not owned by the publisher.

The Hachette Speakers Bureau provides a wide range of authors for speaking events. To find out more, visit hachettespeakersbureau.com or email HachetteSpeakers@hbgusa.com.

Balance books may be purchased in bulk for business, educational, or promotional use. For information, please contact your local bookseller or email the Hachette Book Group Special Markets Department at Special.Markets@hbgusa.com.

Print book interior design by Amy Quinn

Library of Congress Cataloging-in-Publication Data

Name: Levin, Jennifer N., author.
Title: Generation care: the new culture of caregiving / Jennifer N. Levin.
Description: New York, NY: Balance, [2025] | Includes bibliographical references and index.
Identifiers: LCCN 2024040139 | ISBN 9780306832031 (hardcover) |
    ISBN 9780306832048 (trade paperback) | ISBN 9780306832055 (ebook)
Subjects: LCSH: Aging parents—Care—United States. | Chronically Ill—Care—
    United States. | Caregivers—United States—Social conditions. | Caregivers—Services
    for—United States. | Generation Y—United States—Social conditions.
Classification: LCC HQ1063.6 .L487 2025 | DDC 649.8084/60973—dc23/eng/20241221
LC record available at https://lccn.loc.gov/2024040139

ISBNs: 9780306832031(hardcover); 9780306832055 (ebook)

Printed in the United States of America

LSC-C

Printing 1, 2025

To my parents

CONTENTS

NOTE FROM THE AUTHOR

IN RESEARCHING THIS BOOK, I SPOKE WITH CAREGIVERS FROM ALL OVER the United States. Some names used in the book are real, some are not. The caregivers range in age from mid-twenties to early forties and are men and women. (Our generation, of course, also includes nonbinary and transgender people who are caregiving; so far, there's not much research on this demographic. Just because they are not mentioned specifically in this book does not mean they are not included or will not relate to information here; it is also not to refute that they may face additional care obstacles not touched on.)

When I began writing *Generation Care*, I made a commitment to myself that I would introduce each person I interviewed and included here with personal details like their profession or something they like to do; I wouldn't immediately introduce them with the "caregiver" descriptor. I felt it was important to model that the role should not eclipse the person. As I wrote, that changed. I came to believe it was important to keep using the word *caregiver*, to normalize it in relation to the stories of people our age, to band us together under a common title—as different as we and our individual situations might be. I don't want to be misconstrued, so am pointing out this usage as intentional to stress that the experience is shared. Additionally, I don't refer to any of the care recipients by name. It felt most respectful for me not to, since I did not speak with them directly.

This book is intended to give voice to the caregiver experience of people our age in the United States. All direct quotes included are done so with permission; stories from Caregiver Collective, my online support group, have had identities concealed. A caregiver's race, ethnicity, or cultural background is mentioned only when it is relevant to the point being made. These identifiers can absolutely impact our caregiving experience and have meaningful repercussions, from economic impact to resource availability. The length of this book, and its overview approach, allows me only to touch on some of these topics; race and ethnicity play a larger role than I'm able to address here.

Finally, I'd like to make clear: this is an account of the caregiver experience and that includes tough realities and admissions, honestly shared here. Often a caregiver prefaced their remarks by saying, "I feel bad saying this, but for your book—" when they were admitting a harsh reality or complicated emotion. They wanted others *to know*. These admissions are difficult, and I'm grateful to everyone I spoke with for their unshakeable honesty.

This frank discussion should in no way imply that we consider the family member receiving care to be a "burden." They are three-dimensional, dynamic people who we love or, at baseline, in more tumultuous family relationships, feel a familial responsibility to. The burden is the system we care for them under. The burden is the deficit of support available to us and the people we care for. We are all in a difficult situation.

INTRODUCTION

I WASN'T APPREHENSIVE ABOUT TURNING THIRTY, NOT IN THE WAYS movies taught us to be. My mom told me your thirties are the best decade of your life, you know who you *really* are, and I was feeling good at this milestone. I'd established myself in sun-drenched Los Angeles, where I was developing my dream career writing for television and had built a strong network of friends who were my social backbone. I'd recently moved into my first solo apartment, enjoyed being single, and busted my butt putting in long hours to build a career I felt was the right fit for me. On weekends I led an active lifestyle of hiking and paddleboarding and dating melodrama. I came from a stable, albeit divorced, family, with parents whose approval I still sought but whose support I didn't question. I felt fierce and unafraid, the life I was leading felt charmed. A lot had been provided to me; a lot I'd worked hard for.

Then crept in the realization that something was up with my dad. Even with him living across the country in New York, I knew. The guy I spoke with on the phone every day, who was never sick, never not on the go doing his own thing, now in some moments was... *off.* There were falls and worrisome cognitive signs, which evolved into a diagnosis (Parkinson's—wrong) and then another, worse diagnosis (progressive supranuclear palsy, or PSP—bingo) and a move into an assisted living apartment. He was still the same guy, but now with a regimen of pills and regular doctor appointments, physical therapy, and, soon after, a walker for balance. He'd be stubborn and not use the walker to move from his favorite chair to the bathroom or front door, and I'd jump up at the ready to hold him by the arm or I'd pretend it was all cool while I watched with tension. Sometimes when I wasn't fast enough, or wasn't there, he would fall and furniture I grew up with splintered into pieces. Each time I worried that he'd hurt himself but was too proud to admit it.

This intrusion into our lives of something so *medical* was alien, confusing, deeply worrisome; but it was manageable, so I was able to convince myself of false confidence. My father was still in good enough shape that any incidents felt like hiccups we could control, prevent from getting worse. When I was in New York, we still went for regular walks together and out to lunch, we still went to museum exhibits and street fairs.

In February 2013, less than a year after his diagnosis, I was in LA when I received an urgent phone call from my mom: my dad had fallen, this time in his bathroom, where he'd lain for hours until an aide forced themselves in to check on him after he didn't show up for lunch. (Okay: after he didn't show up for lunch, didn't answer any of my calls, and sensing something was wrong, we'd phoned administration and urged them to enter his apartment.) The degenerative brain disease had progressed, his falls now too often and too dangerous, and after a stint in the hospital he'd be transferred to a wheelchair for safety. Immediately, my mind spun with fear about his health getting worse, but I didn't have time to dwell: the assisted living facility dictated that he needed round-the-clock supervision for which he'd need to move into a nursing home...by next week. As the only child of divorced parents, I needed to get home to New York pronto. I booked a flight and spent a whirlwind weekend touring nursing homes with my mom. I quietly cried behind the sunglasses I wore indoors, grappling with every imaginable consideration we needed to address.

Was I prepared? *I was thirty-two.* I hadn't even encountered targeted Instagram ads to freeze my eggs yet.

From then on, the life I'd built for myself was layered with consuming responsibility: I dealt with Medicare, dipped into savings to hire a private nurse's aide, and became my father's healthcare proxy—law now dictated I was the one to make decisions if my dad couldn't. Occasional vacations to New York were replaced by frequent, necessary trips back and forth to handle logistics and keep an eye on my dad's health. I knew he liked me being there, helping him through it, and seeing him gave me peace of mind and comfort. I became his emotional support while I struggled to deal with everything he needed. I monitored the disease's progression: the weakening of his neck muscles, the slowing response of his eye movements, his difficulty swallowing. I quietly agonized watching my father's health deteriorate. His well-being preoccupied my mind; I spent any free moment researching PSP in unrealistic attempts to save him from this disease. My life became a disjointed hybrid of "single-woman problems" and geriatric care.

Becoming my dad's healthcare proxy at a young(ish) age, I felt completely unprepared and alone. Every decision felt like life or death; at times, it was. Meanwhile, his illness took an emotional toll on me that I felt guilty admitting: I was constantly paranoid the other shoe was about to fall, every new symptom and phone call an opportunity for my stomach to drop in fear that this was the worst unraveling. But I also knew it was important to show a brave face, keep spirits up—for me and for my father. The truth? I was full of fear. I dug deep to summon *fierce*, which no longer felt like a personal attribute but a necessity to persevere.

I kept the gritty details, the lonely weight of responsibility, mostly to myself. I was protective of my dad's dignity and didn't want his personality to be eclipsed by the label of "patient" or "victim," which I didn't think he deserved; I used any free time with friends as a mental respite from diagnoses and doctors. Among friends and coworkers, I struggled to project myself as a carefree "has it together" adult, but inwardly I felt like I was crumbling. I didn't think anyone could relate to my new reality of being young and weighted by family illness.

Why would I? Millennials (born 1981–1996, of which I'm one) had a pretty shit reputation at the time. Countless headlines and commentators deemed us an entitled, selfish generation: young adults who sponged off our parents, still lived in their homes because our latte spending was out of hand. Our resistance to fiscal responsibility left us inadequate to be self-sufficient, or at best, unwilling. Millennials, it was known, didn't want to work for anyone; we wanted to be entrepreneurs, CEOs of our own destiny—and we'd let our parents fund us until we got there.

The stereotype was antithetical to the hard-working and debt-laden reality of people I knew who were my age; but it was so widely accepted that, for years, from the time I was in my twenties through my mid-thirties, many people my age refused to identify themselves as Millennials. The bias turned us against each other, prevented us from associating with our generation, and painted a portrait that didn't align with how we knew we were living. Still, when comparing knowledge of my friends' lives to my own, I barely knew anyone else my age going through something similar to what I was living with my dad.

In 2015, the same year the *Washington Post* published "Five Really Good Reasons to Hate Millennials" (thanks), Easter Seals and Mass Mutual offered a sober reality check: over ten million Millennials in the United States were already caregiving for ill or ailing family members. The report floored me. It was a year after my dad passed and I was still processing what had happened; this was the first time I realized, "Wait a minute, that's me." Until I read that study, I didn't even know that I fell into the "caregiver" category. I thought caregivers were paid professionals, nurses' aides, or—the typical media portrayal—an older woman caring for geriatric parents; I was just being a good daughter. Not to mention, I wasn't living with my dad, helping him 24/7, so how could this caregiver title apply to me? The report demystified the role, which can entail everything from doling out medication and arranging doctor appointments to changing colostomy bags—and not just for parents but also for siblings, spouses, and grandparents. I couldn't believe how many of my peers were also going through this intense rite of passage, how widespread the situation was (at the time, nearly 1 in 4 people aged 18–33 was a caregiver). But if I wasn't alone, why did I feel so isolated? Why wasn't anyone talking about it?

I wrote an article for *Cosmopolitan* ("I Became My Father's Parent at 32") that revealed my experience and the surprising statistic of my caregiving peers. It was the first time I outed myself as a caregiver. I was terrified. Millennials acting as unpaid family caregivers wasn't in the public discourse, and in black and white, I'd served up family details that for years I'd kept private. The decision to go public was the key to the connection I'd needed. Almost immediately, young adults from across the country began contacting me. Peers I'd grown up with and people I'd never met confided that they'd experienced the same thing but had never told anyone; friends were surprised to learn I'd had an ailing parent at all. People who had never before felt like a peer understood them finally had someone to relate to, including me. In DMs and emails, we began trading histories, and I felt connected to strangers I instantly shared a shorthand with. Finally, the conversation had started.

I knew there was more to be done. All the support groups I found were tailored to Boomer caregivers; no group focused on caregivers our age and how differently we meet the challenge, or addressed the emotional circumstances of facing this at a younger age than anticipated. I didn't understand why, in the face of a loved one's illness, anyone our age should need to reinvent the wheel in figuring out *how* to provide care, or feel so alone doing it. Together we could share not only support but also resources, the practical advice hard won. In the article's wake I created Caregiver Collective, an online community for Millennials (and perennially left out Gen Xers and those not-yet-acknowledged in Gen Z) experiencing family caregiving, the first of its kind. And the most amazing thing happened—

People joined.

Millennials from all over the country began sharing personal stories, many for the first time; I could practically feel the weight lifting from their shoulders as they finally admitted their reality. Moderating the message board, every day I read firsthand accounts of what others are truly experiencing. Those who are too shy confide in me directly.

Through Caregiver Collective, I met and still meet incredible people and can see just how varied our generation's caregiver experience is: we're almost fifty-fifty along gender lines and ethnically diverse. There's no archetype of who we are; we're everyone. We care for the family we're legally or biologically related to as well as "chosen" family, like neighbors and friends. Some members, like me, find themselves providing care suddenly and for an intense stint; others have been caring for family most of their lives with no change in sight. We connect through the shared experience, are cognizant that it is a defining role, but avoid being singularly defined by it. There is more we want for ourselves in our young(ish) lives.

Here are a few of the people I've come to know (their stories are real but some names have been changed). You may have met them at the office or at a mutual friend's birthday party; if you asked how they were, they'd probably have said, "Fine, thanks!" Here's honesty:

From the first online support chat she joined, Michelle and I hit it off as native New Yorkers who happened to have grown up in adjacent neighborhoods. In her early thirties, she's the only child of Chinese American parents, single, and is interested in dating but has no idea how to meet someone while caring for her mom, who has chronic kidney disease. She works full-time in experiential design and turned down a job relocation offer abroad to remain home:

> I've been caregiving for fifteen years and I've been cooped up with my parents, one of whom I am caregiving for, for the past pandemic year. It's hard to be stuck in an environment in which you are constantly reminded that your needs come last because you're not the sick one.... I've struggled to have an identity apart from being a daughter/caregiver, and I've found that I even struggle to articulate what I actually want or feel because everything I do is so instinctively grounded in the perspective of what is best for the family.

John was one of the first people to join Caregiver Collective. Before his parents required care, John had a job in politics and was enrolled in a graduate program in New Jersey, where he's from. We first spoke off-board three years ago, when I interviewed him for an article I was writing. John can be counted on to be a supportive presence in the group, always reminding people to maintain their own interests outside of caregiving:

> *I'm thirty-five and have been a full-time caregiver to my parents for five years after they had strokes within a month of each other. I feel like I've worked harder than I did when I was in the mainstream workforce. I've felt isolated from those my age because of my responsibilities. I feel as though not many people my age understand....I don't know if people realize how difficult the choices we've made are, often with no substantial support.*

Brandon is one of three brothers. He's into creative writing, struggled to quit smoking, and a few years ago moved from New York to Michigan to live with his mom, who has Parkinson's and fibromyalgia and can't live alone. He's the only one of his siblings to assume care. He often joined Zoom Support Chats from his garage, the only place he could find privacy:

> *I've been doing this about three years, half of that full-time, and still trying to find a way to balance my life in more. It'll surprise me, sometimes, how far I got from my old life in such little time. Like, I'll go out for a walk in the city on a rare night to myself, and see people with their friends, hanging out outside a bar or something, and it'll be like, "Whoa, yeah, I used to just grab my coat and go meet up with people, unplanned."*

Isolation from peers and friends was a recurring theme among Collective members—but far from the only one. It wasn't long before I began to see many patterns: the fear of losing a job when you're caring for a loved one before you've established a strong employment or savings history, the debilitating emotional stress of caring for a parent before you've built a family of your own, the fear that you'll never have even a piece of what you dreamt for your own life...and feeling guilty for even thinking about it. You don't hear concerns like this in the average support group of people who began caring later in life, after they had a chance to establish themselves; these are the deep-seated worries gnawing at those of us with a long road ahead. Unless you're in a group of like-minded people, these feelings may not get expressed at all.

Before she joined Caregiver Collective, Mia tried attending support groups at the local VA. In her thirties, she's the primary caregiver for her best friend, a veteran her age who sustained severe injuries. The experience of searching for support left her feeling even more isolated. The veteran support groups she attended were for Vietnam-era families, and local caregiver groups were filled with seniors who excluded her for being younger and, they assumed, a bit green. She described how finding our group provided an assuring sense of community; she was boosted by the articles and caregiving resources members share to help each other.

The solution-oriented and optimistic approach of Caregiver Collective that Mia mentioned is something I, too, hadn't witnessed in other caregiver groups. I realized that, through this communion of voices, I was gaining amazing insight into our collective experience. Meanwhile, I observed the far-reaching impact caregiving was having (and will continue to have) on our generation: economically, mentally, physically, and the list goes on. It's heightened for us to a level I didn't anticipate but that we can't ignore.

Caregiving is a familial reality that has occurred for eons, so why are Millennials experiencing it more acutely than previous generations? The answer doesn't lie solely with the passing of time and evolution of society; I learned that even when caregiving simultaneously with our Boomer counterparts, the repercussions on Millennials—like being demoted or fired from work—are harsher. So: *WTF*.

That's when I got in deep. I pored over economic and employment statistics, medical-leave policies, and personal caregiving stories from peers. I realized caregiving isn't just happening *to* us but historical and cultural influences are leading us to confront the issue in new ways. Caregiving impacts how our families operate today, and it will impact how our families look in the future. I was getting a great sense of our big picture of care and insights into how our generation was living when the global pandemic turned everything on its head.

Coronavirus rocked every aspect of our lives, particularly for those of us with high-risk family members, and cast a spotlight on our country's care crisis. The curtain was pulled back to reveal the impossible balancing act families across the country were barely managing between paid employment and the demands of home care work. Working moms drew most of the focus, but the pandemic also initiated a larger national dialogue around those of us caregiving—finally, at a time when its intensity had ramped up and fewer outside resources were available. The combination eroded personal boundaries and put the gaping holes of our healthcare system on full display. People began talking about caregivers; people began realizing *they already were caregivers* in ways they hadn't recognized before. There was a noticeable uptick in Caregiver Collective membership; for the first time, many new members were young adults speculating on their aging parents' increasing needs. More Millennials became aware of the vulnerability of their family.

Then, during the pandemic's first wave, President Biden announced an infrastructure plan that acknowledged family caregiving as part of the backbone necessary for our country's operation; his proposal addressed concerns (ahem, *needs*) that had become touchy for caregivers, after decades of being dismissed. It didn't go over well. *Is care a part of national infrastructure?* was a question not just discussed but hotly debated; the question sparked controversy that lit up nightly news programs and weekly op-eds. Millennials, who provide so much of the care that goes unnoticed beyond our own families, found themselves in the crosshairs of controversial government policy. The need for our nation to understand our culture of care became more apparent than ever.

This book explains the damaging effects our country's existing care crisis has had on our generation and how it happened, told through statistical research and personal experiences. I interviewed dozens of Millennials caught in the care crosshairs who were ready to talk; you'll hear their stories and mine. We'll explore how the Millennial attitude toward family leads us to meet the caregiving challenge differently. We'll discuss how national and world events both exacerbated our care emergency and pulled it into sharp focus along with the changed landscape of how our country thinks about health and sickness. But this book, at the intersection of realism and optimism, also shares what we can do about it—critical conversations to have today *and* tangible solutions for our future.

I'm now in my early forties, and I can say with certainty that my thirties *did* define who I *really* am—and revealed to me a shared experience of my generation, one that connects us in unforeseen ways and continues to shape the adults we've become. When I began writing this book, the Millennials I spoke to felt like no one understood how the caregiving experience, so outside of their control, changed their entire lives in an instant, how it halted their own plans indefinitely, and added heaps of uncertainty. The pandemic we all lived through opened the possibility for larger understanding of how common it is for us to compromise personal advancement for the care of our families, how so often it doesn't feel like a choice but a necessity. Moving forward, these lessons can go beyond explaining individual circumstances; they can help shape a broader infrastructure to support our nation's health. We need societal systems that work with us and how we're living, not a system our generation must awkwardly struggle to conform to for survival. These are issues not only for Millennials but also for the Gen X caregivers who silently live this crisis with us and the many Gen Z caregivers already following in our wake.

I hope that if you are living this experience or already have, you find yourself in these pages. I know you are physically exhausted and emotionally depleted, but I hope you recognize you are part of a movement with heart and connection at its very core. The ways we care for family, and each other, define our generation and ourselves.

So, are you ready? Let's have an honest discussion about the care we provide.

PART ONE

HERE WE ARE

CHAPTER 1

WHO WE ARE:
A SNAPSHOT

"CAN I JUST RUN AWAY?"

This was my oldest friend Amy on the phone with me one evening. I was thirty-two at the time, she was thirty-one, and earlier that day we'd toured a nursing home together, each evaluating it for our respective fathers—very different from the Barbie Dreamhouses that occupied our afternoons decades earlier. My dad needed to move out of assisted living right away; Amy was in a longer process of moving her father from a rehab facility in Florida back to New York, where she lived and would be able to manage his care more easily. Amy was planning her wedding while knee-deep in this nursing home research—which she just learned she'd have to throw in the mental dumpster: her eighty-four-year-old dad, who weeks earlier had had a stroke, informed her he wouldn't be leaving Florida. The reason? He'd just paid a matchmaker $15,000.

Running away, it seemed, was her only viable next step. Would she actually do it? Of course not. Probably not. But if an electronic boardwalk genie offered to grant her a wish, I think running away would be top of mind. The whole situation was so frustrating for her...infuriating, even. And just so, so...*ridiculous.* It was also a snapshot of the Millennial experience.

I'VE BEEN WRITING THIS BOOK FOR A FEW YEARS NOW, AND BEFORE THIS have published articles on the topic of Millennial family caregivers. In this work I often face a common uphill battle: when I tell people what I'm writing about, that caregivers in our generation number in the millions and there's a need to build awareness and support for us, I notice…how do I phrase this?

They don't really believe me.

Countless times, I detect skepticism about how prevalent the issue is, despite sharing my own family experience, national statistics, and how active my online support group is. Every person takes convincing.

For me, this is frustrating. Infuriating, even. Faced with evidence, why are people so skeptical to hear Millennials step up en masse to provide family care? Most likely because we don't fit neatly into the box of who people imagine someone in that role to be; we're not the caregiver archetype you immediately picture. A lot of this confusion stems from who we believe caregivers to be, and how that's antithetical to what we think about Millennials. We need to come to terms with the realities of both and where they intersect.

I WAS BORN IN 1981, WHICH MAKES ME A "GERIATRIC MILLENNIAL" TO ANYone who wants to royally piss me off. But whether you were born in 1980 or 1996, we're a part of the largest living generation in the United States, 72.19 million strong.[1] Our generation got its name because our eldest entered adulthood around the turn of the millennium; we have seen some shit.

Millennials were raised on the notion that a successful career follows a college education. As a result, we were more likely to pursue higher education than previous generations.[2] Those of us who attended college or beyond took on unprecedented student loan debt to do it. We graduated into a job market that was fucked, worse for some of us than for others. A 2010 publication by Pew Research deemed our generation "Confident. Connected. Open to Change";[3] ten years later the *Washington Post* crowned us "The unluckiest generation in U.S. history."[4]

Evidently, by summer 2020, when that *Washington Post* article was written, a lot had changed. Along with the global pandemic and tanking economy, the media cycle was also ready to admit that the average Millennial—maligned for years by US media and pop culture—had not been dealt the entitlement hand like the world had been led to believe. We've experienced slower economic growth since entering the workforce than any other generation in US history. We've faced three recessions, each with the capacity to decrease our savings and life expectancy (this is based on research and not a flair for drama). We've lived through and have been shaped by Columbine, homeland terror, opioid addictions, and the COVID-19 pandemic. We've evolved with the internet; we now have dogs and babies with their own Instagram handles. Now let's square all of this with who a *caregiver* is.

WHEN I REFERENCE *CAREGIVERS* IN THIS BOOK, I'M DISCUSSING AN *informal* or *family caregiver*. This is a person who provides care for a family member or friend who needs help caring for themselves, such as elderly, chronically ill, disabled, or mentally ill persons. (Although I don't directly address it in this book, some caregivers provide care for people with substance abuse and addiction problems—to call this a big issue in our country is an understatement.) Care responsibilities can range from buying groceries and preparing meals to administering home medical care. Caregiving can come on suddenly, with a major medical incident such as a stroke or terminal diagnosis, or is a role someone slides into gradually as the needs and dependence of the person needing care increase. Some caregivers live with the family member they care for; others visit them in their homes or live-in facilities.

In the United States today, there are over fifty-three million family caregivers.[5] In 2018, over ten million of them were Millennials—since then, the number has only surged. Why are so many people providing family care? Because our country, as it stands today, can't function without this "free" labor.

To operate, the US healthcare system relies on unpaid family caregivers. It's sneaky business born from (hopefully) good intentions: when someone is living with a chronic condition (anything from cancer to neurological conditions such as Alzheimer's and dementia), if they are not hospitalized for in-patient care, they are sent home. So far, sounds okay; an overwhelming majority of Americans want to age at home.[6] But these people still require treatment and care, and the US system leaves the family to assume the responsibility of figuring that out. With the exorbitant cost of paid care (like in-home aides and living facilities), often care duties are taken on by blindsided family or even friends. It's a massive undertaking, requiring time, money, organization, and emotional energy. In 2021, family caregivers accounted for $600 billion in unpaid labor.[7] (I'll let you read that number again.) This was up from $470 billion in 2017. The value of unpaid family care exceeds that of paid home care and is increasing in economic value.

The pandemic added 1.2 million more disabled people to the population, and worsened the (already pressing) shortage of professional caregivers, necessitating more hours and higher intensity of care by family.[8] The caregiving workforce is expected to expand but still contends with the challenges of high turnover (40–60 percent each year), low pay, and insufficient training.[9] The professional home care shortage is a serious, serious issue. By shifting the responsibility of family care primarily to relatives and friends, it has created a care crisis and one we are not climbing out of anytime soon: the United States is on track to "run out" of family caregivers as the aging population outpaces those available to (one day) provide care.[10] As of today, no federal solutions in place are able to fully deal with this crisis.

WHY ARE THERE SO MANY OF US?

Sixty percent of first-time caregivers are Millennials or in Gen Z. A significant number of us took on the role during the pandemic.[11] Millennials aren't just members of the caregiving population; our generation is being impacted in unprecedented ways: we are caring earlier and in larger numbers than ever before. We are a huge indicator of where the care crisis is going; many of us are already there.

Why are there more of us now than ever? Boomers and their elders are aging during a time when modern medicine allows people to live longer, in general and with chronic illness, and at home. Also, since September 11, our generation has had its fair share of returning veterans, which put young adults into the position of caring for a spouse or a sibling very early in adulthood. Long COVID now adds more caregivers to our ranks.

I also believe the Millennial mindset plays a role in our inclination to personally assume costly family care duties, despite the fact that we are financially less well off than previous generations. We were raised with role models like Doogie Howser, MD, a teenager who legally performed surgeries, and the Goonies, who endangered themselves to save their family homes from development monsters when their parents couldn't afford to. We were presented with economic and medical realities and it was the kids' responsibility to fix them, to be the adults in the room. My observation is not hyperbole: cultural research shows that Millennials feel responsibility to others first, and to ourselves second[12]—just think of the rise of socially conscious businesses in our generation. Many of us also have closer relationships with our parents than previous generations did. This is the stuff that shapes our tendency to personally handle their care, no matter the weight of the responsibility. With so many of us taking on caregiving, our generation's mindset has changed what family care looks like and who engages in it.

I SEE YOU: A SNAPSHOT

To paint a clearer picture, here's a snapshot of Millennial caregivers based on research by AARP and the National Alliance for Caregiving. For those of you who feel like an outlier to your generation, I think you'll find yourself here—and find that archetypes are broken.

We Have a More Complex Face Than Previous Generations

For the first time, caregivers of our generation are almost equally men and women. Like Millennials in general, Millennial caregivers are ethnically diverse; more than half are people of color, including Black Americans, Latinx, Asian Americans, and Pacific Islanders.[13] A greater proportion of Millennial caregivers identify as LGBTQ+ than in previous generations of caregivers, and they care for relatives and, often, "chosen" family.

We're Busting Our Butts

Millennials are more likely to balance hourly work or careers with caregiving compared to older generations. On average, in addition to our jobs, Millennials provide enough hours of unpaid care per week (approximately twenty-five) for it to be considered a part-time job.[14] One in four provides care for forty hours a week or more, equivalent to a full-time job.[15] Half of us are the sole informal caregiver, and even fewer of us have any paid help (compared to caregivers older than us). In general, we earn below the national median and are financially strained.[16] The care we provide comes out of our bank accounts, whether in lost wages or out-of-pocket care expenses. We more often report financial repercussions resulting from caregiving, like paying bills late, taking on debt, and not being able to afford basic expenses.

Who We Care For

The majority of us are caring for parents or grandparents, but the spectrum of our care recipients includes spouses, siblings, children with disabilities, and "chosen family" (friends or neighbors who need care).[17] Millennials are more likely than other generations to care for someone with a mental health or emotional issue (33 percent of us); these caregivers (in general) report even higher emotional stress levels than other caregivers.[18] Because we begin so young, our generation may be caregiving for decades longer than our elders.

We Are Now Multigenerational Caregivers

About 30 percent of all family caregivers in the United States are "sandwich generation" caregivers who care for an older adult and children in the same house. These caregivers are now more likely to be Millennials or Gen Z.[19] This statistic does not include the caregivers our age who are caring for a spouse, sibling, or other relationship while also raising kids; these are the multigenerational caregivers (caring for at least two family members of different generations) that we'll bring into focus later in this book. Multigen caregivers redefine our traditional understanding of the sandwich generation and are often left out of the conversation—until now.

We Provide a Range of Care

More than half of Millennial caregivers perform complex activities of daily living (ADLs) and medical/nursing tasks.[20] ADLs include helping the person you care for to bathe, eat, use the bathroom, or transfer (for example, move from their wheelchair to the bed or the toilet). Medical or nursing tasks can include wound care and helping with home medical equipment. People interviewed for this book spoke about responsibilities like performing daily dialysis at home (which requires thorough sterilization beforehand) and changing colostomy bags. Fewer than one-third of the Millennials performing these tasks received instruction on *how*. Nearly all Millennials providing care help with one or more household tasks, such as giving medications, managing finances, and prepping meals. I was my father's healthcare proxy, meaning I was legally responsible for making his healthcare decisions if he couldn't.

Our Health Sucks

Yes, we are young, but care takes a physical and mental health toll that is quantifiable and backed by research. A greater proportion of caregiving Millennials report being in "fair or poor health" as compared to other generations, and the emotional stress we report from care is "moderate to high."[21] This stress has been shown to lead to negative coping mechanisms in our generation, such as alcohol abuse or smoking, and an alarming rate of suicide ideation during the pandemic. In addition, Millennials are among those least likely to have health insurance; financial and time strains translate into cutting back on our own doctor appointments and preventative care.[22]

We Find Positive Value in Providing Care

Millennials are more likely to report that they've experienced emotional benefits from providing care, such as spending more time with a family member they love and increased emotional intimacy. Finding positive value in family care work has been shown in studies to be key to building resilience when our role is through. In speaking with caregivers of different generations, I have noticed that, on the whole, Millennials take an optimistic and solution-oriented approach.

HOW WE EXPERIENCE CAREGIVING DIFFERENTLY

Millennial caregivers have taken on care in the formative years when we're expected, and hoping, to build our "adult" lives. We are in our family-building era, yet caregiving can dictate whether we're able to marry, have children, or even date. We may grieve the lives we "thought" we'd have.

Taking on care at a younger age than we're prepared for creates new complications and gives rise to dire consequences. For the many people who haven't yet started families of their own, it may be their first time shouldering responsibility and care for someone else, and there is a steep learning curve. Feelings that they've taken on the role prematurely, and without peer modeling, results in younger adults caring in silence and handling everything alone, as well as experiencing increased isolation from friends and colleagues. The stress of balancing the various parts of their lives that hold significant weight at this age (such as building employment history and financial earnings, their social life) with care results in younger caregivers experiencing higher "caregiver burden" than older caregivers.[23] (A note: I don't know anyone who likes the term *caregiver burden*, myself included, but it's the official term for a studied stress experience, so I'll use it throughout the book.)

Compounding the isolation and exaggerating the learning curve, Millennials frequently don't identify with the term *caregiver*. There are many reasons for this, including lack of awareness of the role. Multiple people interviewed for this book considered themselves caregivers once they were in their twenties or thirties but, upon reflection, realized their care responsibilities began much earlier (as a teenager or even a child); because their role built progressively, they hadn't previously identified as caregivers, although they were already living it. Some caregivers act in support of the "primary" caregiver (meaning they are not the point person and don't take on all the duties themselves), so don't realize the title applies to them as well. Other caregivers don't think of what they contribute as caregiving, particularly when the work fulfills more of a coordinator role. In a hypothetical example, Mike's father has early-onset dementia and needs round-the-clock supervision. Mike's relationship with his dad is not great, and he knows he's not equipped to provide this level of care at home. Mike coordinates moving his father into an assisted living facility with memory care: it requires research, tours, coordinating whether insurance will pay for it or, if not, who will. A big move of Dad's things out of his house is also on Mike's to-do list. Mike may not realize it, but this book is for him, too. He's been doing care work.

Millennials also approach the healthcare system differently: we're skeptical because we've seen enough to believe it's profits over people; because of our age, some of us have found we're not taken seriously by doctors; and we're digital natives seeking online access. We take things into our own hands.

All these generational factors shape our care experiences. Lack of understanding of our generation's role in caregiving—whether misunderstood by others or ourselves—is one root of our greater issue as care providers and as individuals. The experiential knowledge and day-to-day of caregivers our age are often overlooked, and we are left at the mercy of a system that fails to meet the care crisis where we are and how we are caring.

CHAPTER 2

IDENTITY CRISIS AND CAREGIVING IN SILENCE

When you live with and care for somebody who is sick, and in our case, chronically sick, their needs are kind of always priority.... It seeps into how you even start to think about things....

I realized, whenever people asked me what I wanted to do or what I liked, I immediately would position it from the perspective of what our family likes or what our family needed. And I'm just like: Oh wait, what do I want? It takes active effort on my part to even start to identify that.... It gets to a point where it's almost like second nature [to] think about theirs as your own. And when people asked me how I was doing, I'd be like, "Oh, my mom's doing great, so I'm doing pretty great too." Or like, "She's kind of shitty right now, so not so great for me." It would always be in relation [to] that.

—Michelle, 31

CAREGIVERS OUR AGE, AND OF OUR GENERATION, FACE AN IDENTITY crisis. There's a crisis of self, when your personal interests, maybe not even fully developed yet, are pushed aside for the benefit of the person you care for, or because there just isn't any time between work and care. Each caregiver interviewed for this book was asked what they like to do for fun. A handful couldn't answer the question. They didn't know or couldn't remember. (One even told me he'd ask his best friend later that day, "He must know.")

There's a crisis of caregiver identity, when you don't relate to the term. If you don't think the title applies to you, you don't self-identify with this group. This can prohibit seeking or accessing available resources or advocating for yourself.

There's a crisis among peers, when you feel like an outlier because of your caregiver role and don't relate to the lives of your friends or people you know. You may no longer relate to your own life outside of caregiving, which is particularly disconcerting.

These identity crises prevent us from being our authentic selves, from forming connections with others. They keep us quiet, feeling like, *No one will relate, so what's the use?* The identity disconnect keeps us from getting the support we need, which might be within reach, but our hands are clamped over our mouths.

Finally, there's an identity crisis of our generation when our culture of care battles directly against that well-worn Millennial reputation we talked about. This isn't so much among people our age but some people of older generations without frank knowledge of our realities who undermine the difficulty of our experience. The identity crisis hinders efforts to address the caregivers our age who need help, whether by reaching out to them for emotional and logistical support or considering them in caregiver policies.

"I'M NOT A CAREGIVER"

Over half of people providing family care in the United States do not self-identify as caregivers, and there's been some research into why this is.[1] A lot of caregivers are like me: I was plain ignorant of what a caregiver is; I thought they were professional aides. I was my dad's *daughter*, doing what a daughter does. I was spending time with him because I wanted to, and when he needed something, I helped him. That was my frame of mind, even knowing the toll it took on me was different than I had ever experienced before his illness. According to a study by the National Family Caregivers Association and the National Alliance for Caregiving, it's common for caregivers of all ages to associate the word with a paid professional, mostly because they feel the term lacks the warmth and love involved with caring for a family member.[2]

And that's another reason: some people just don't like the term *caregiver*. At the time of the study, the term *family caregiver* was better received by those providing care, but overall people were unsure of how to use the moniker so...didn't. How can you normalize a role when people won't say the word because they didn't "get" it? Some caregivers, even when they know they are one, don't want to identify with the term because it feels like a group they don't want to be part of, that the label will overshadow their other selves and define them. (In some scenarios, this unfortunately can be true: unconscious bias of employers toward employees, or potential employees, they know are caregiving is a very real thing that can result in discrimination and exclusion.) Others don't want to give the role a name at all because, similar to my previous sentiment, it's "what families do." Sometimes someone is not the primary caregiver and doesn't feel right adopting the title knowing someone else is more "boots on the ground," despite knowing how much they themselves contribute. When you are a younger caregiver, there are even more reasons you may not self-identify as one.

The media image we have of an unpaid family caregiver in the United States looks nothing like us: an older woman (in media representations I grew up with: white), maybe already a retiree, who is caring for an elderly parent. This archetype taken as a definition prevents both younger people and men from identifying with the role. Particularly for our generation, in which men comprise almost half of those already caring, this is a big one. "Men were actually really quite harmed by the gender norms related to caregiving, in that it's harder for them to ask for help, it's harder for them to actually get the support that they need to do what is a very emotionally challenging—and otherwise [difficult]—thing to do," renowned labor leader and caregiver advocate Ai-jen Poo told Bustle.[3] Caring Across Generations, the organization for which she serves as director, began the #WeKnowYouCare campaign to bring visibility to male caregivers.

Sometimes we don't identify with the role because we don't even realize we're living it, particularly when its responsibilities begin subtly.

About half of the caregivers I interviewed for this book told me that, in retrospect, they began caregiving at a much younger age than they had initially realized, that the role had begun well before they considered themselves "caregivers." In most of these cases, they adopted the title after a major incident occurred, like a bad fall or major diagnosis, and their loved one's needs intensified. Only looking back do they realize they had already been assisting and accommodating that person's health needs for years; sometimes they even realized it in the course of our conversation.

"I'M NOT ONE OF *THOSE* MILLENNIALS"

After enough confrontations I hit a point where I had to wonder why, even today, some people remain skeptical that caregiving impacts our generation the way it does. Truth is, the outdated Millennial reputation still—ridiculously—plays a role. Some people are reluctant to identify with other Millennials, despite a shared experience; others hear "Millennial" still as a synonym for "young and entitled." When I first began research for this book, a high school friend asked why I focused so much on Millennials, her facial expression the equivalent of a gag reflex. "Because we are Millennials," I answered.

"No," she protested. "Millennials are *the worst*."

When I backed up my argument by naming the year we were both born, which is widely regarded as the advent of the generation, she dismissed it.

"Fine," she said. "But I'm not one of *those* Millennials."

I felt like I was having this conversation in a time warp, but the reality is some people still subscribe to this and refuse to identify with the generation. If you're a caregiver this age who still believes this about your peers, it can foster feelings of being an outlier; it can lead people to assume caregiving might not touch this generation at all.

In another recent conversation, a woman I'd just met who was closer to my mom's demo thought my book topic was interesting but couldn't understand how caregiving was enough of an issue for our generation to necessitate conversation. For one, she said, Millennials are young, presumably far too young for our parents to be an age that requires care. (I faced this same incorrect assumption at a national caregiving conference I attended.) And second, she said, Millennials are greedy and lazy. She went on to tell me about the young Millennial women among her son's friends who were unwilling to work and instead date men for their money. It fit neatly into the old Millennial trope. Her subjective retelling was problematic for a lot of reasons, but I'll narrow it to one: the women she was talking about were twenty years old, too young to be Millennials no matter what they were or weren't up to. When I corrected her mistake, she was confused that Millennials could be my age, just over forty. Some people still don't realize Millennials have aged and we didn't deserve the derisive reputation in the first place.

As we've gotten older, our reputation among most, thankfully, has adjusted to our reality. I recently saw it summed up nicely online in a TikTok video of two middle-aged men laughing hysterically, flailing around in hysterical fits beneath a spinning UFO, which hovers above them. The caption reads: "POV: Millennials when aliens arrive to be our final trauma." What our generation has lived through as we entered adulthood, and through it to date, has been well documented. Millennials are tired from the multiple economic and world crises that kicked off when the eldest of us were in our twenties. When we first entered the zeitgeist, we were the young generation rising up; now a lot of us are parents whose kids participate in active shooter drills. All of us are in therapy or need it but can't afford it. At this point, declaring yourself a Millennial feels more like a Census answer than a judgment call. A recent Instagram post asked, "Remember when being a Millennial meant we were young?"

Still there remains some holdover of the crappy Millennial reputation, one that prevents people from believing Millennials would take on the caregiver role, or any hardship, and do so in such large numbers.

"I'M NOT TALKING ABOUT IT"

Despite millions of us experiencing it, few of us disclose our caregiving reality. We soak up the curated social media lives of others, which contributes to our perceived isolation, and paint our own social image to gloss over the difficult reality. Maybe we choose to relate over other chaotic shared experiences: noisy politics, increased crime, a heatwave. Expressing exhaustion for any of these is common practice. But when it comes to care, people close to us, and the country, remain in the dark about what is actually going on.

I didn't disclose much about my dad's illness or how I was providing care because I was protective of his identity. My dad had a level of vanity I admired: he was always well-groomed, haircut sharp; even his jeans were tailored. Throughout my life, including when he was in the nursing home, he always changed for dinner, always ran a comb through his hair before seeing anyone. My cousin recently said, "I always remember your dad's shoes." He kept each pair pristine, polished, and well cared for. Laces were given careful attention so they laid flat. The man was a perfectionist, and his appearance was no exception. I didn't want to tell my friends how many shirts he went through a day now that he was drooling during meals; how utensils had become difficult so food inevitably fell into his lap or hit the floor. How much energy I'd watch him exert to lift his chin from his chest so he could look me in the eyes and smile or laugh at a joke. I wasn't embarrassed, and I don't think he was either, but I didn't want these new developments to steal attention from who he was. I didn't want people to mistake it for weakness. I was grieving the changes I was seeing and probably didn't want to admit they were happening. In retrospect, with a bit more maturity, I don't think my dad would've cared if I did, and I don't think it would've made a difference to anyone who really knew him. And yet, so much was changing then and so much felt out of my control, somehow it became another insecurity for me.

Ron, a man in his early forties who has been providing care and financial assistance to his mom since he was about fourteen years old, said that he kept caregiving a secret for years. His mother is bipolar with psychosis, now also in the initial stages of dementia, and is prone to psychotic episodes. For a long time, Ron's silence wasn't so much a decision as an unconscious pattern; he just figured caregiving was his responsibility and obligation. There was also a component of shame. It was in the workplace that he picked up on his own reasons for staying quiet:

> *I think a lot of it was to appear, I don't want to say "normal," but yeah…*
> *to fit into the group, your peer group. And you want to seem like everyone*
> *else, right?…It wasn't like this conscious withholding, initially. It was just*
> *more like, nobody else deals with this stuff, so why would I bring this up?…*
> *Nobody's talking about taking care of parents.…So I think that was sort of*
> *just the way I dealt with it. I don't think it was intentional withholding, I*
> *think it was more a desire to be seen and to relate.*

In recent years Ron has begun to voice with honesty that he is a caregiver and what his responsibilities are at home. He realized there were others "suffering in silence" to connect with. He sees it as a major component to living authentically and being true to himself. There's a lesson in this: as a guest on Brené Brown's podcast, Surgeon General Vivek Murthy stated that not being "true to yourself" is what loneliness (and thus, isolation) is born of. Caregivers our age experience loneliness en masse (we'll dig into this later), so Ron is on the right track. Any shame for his family situation that Ron felt when he was younger has undergone revision:

> *Once I was able to realize, "Holy crap are you kidding, Ron? There's absolutely no shame in what you're trying to do and the situation you're thrust*
> *into," it's really just for the better.…In terms of my value system, I value*
> *authenticity because I saw how hard it was to connect with others without*
> *being your truest self.…*
>
> *The thing I would always want people to know is that there is no shame in*
> *acknowledging that this experience colors your vision and the lens on which*
> *you see everything in your life. And that's okay because that's your story and*
> *that's your journey. You're better for it.*

Kaci, a teacher in her late thirties who has been providing care for her mom since her mid-twenties, felt the ostracization Ron described—it got worse when she participated in caregiver support groups:

It took me a long time to be able to identify as a caregiver....I think part of it, too, was finding the group of Millennial caregivers because it was so hard. Sometimes I went to the Working Daughter[4] stuff for a while, but then I was like, I feel like I'm in a totally different spot in my life. I didn't get to have kids. I didn't get to get married. I didn't get to hit those milestones. It was also hard because I was in groups with people whose parents were dying all the time, and that really stressed me constantly to see everyone's obituaries on Facebook.

Kaci is not the only caregiver our age who told me they felt worse after attending a caregiver support group; seeking the mutual support of people in the same boat, they instead were met with people much older than they were, which underscored feelings of being an outlier (it's one of the reasons I began Caregiver Collective, but let's not consider this the only takeaway of attending a broader support group, which we'll talk more about later).

HOW CAREGIVING INFLUENCES OUR PERSONAL IDENTITIES

We don't just perceive a disconnect with peers, we can also feel an uncomfortable internal disconnect when confronted with our former selves— our lives before caregiving. Alexandra, whose mom had glioblastoma, packed up her life in Thailand as a travel blogger and moved back home to care for her mom in upstate New York. Before her mom's brain cancer, Alex was living a "jetsetter lifestyle," and the switch to quiet domesticity was jarring. Traveling to New York City for a quick personal break underscored how different her life had become.

Michelle, on the other hand, felt so consumed by care for her mom, who had renal disease, that she used her "other" life for escapism and a reorientation to her self. Her career became a coping mechanism and she leaned into being a workaholic.

It's not only anecdotal: a study found that loss of identity comes about as a result of engulfment in the caregiver role and was found to be more common among younger caregivers (also among female caregivers and caregiving spouses).[5] Limited social contact and lack of social roles outside of caregiving (like no longer connecting with friends, limited dating or relationships, compromised or eliminated work relationships) were found to be related to greater loss of self. The loss of self is, no surprise, related to lower self-esteem and greater depressive symptoms.

Michelle found that in social situations it became difficult for her to differentiate herself from caregiving. She didn't know how to talk about herself without talking about her care, even to people she didn't know. At a certain point, she realized that if she met someone casually at a one-off event, like a virtual mixer or networking evening, she didn't need to mention caregiving. She had to coach herself not to bring up her mom's care, psych herself into it, and said she swung from one extreme to the other: from not knowing how *not* to bring it up to not mentioning it all—which she found just as uncomfortable:

> *You feel like you're hiding something even though you're not, just because it is so much part of your everyday. It's almost like you're putting a mask on to enjoy this time and then go back to your life.*

When speaking to people familiar with her family situation, Kaci finds her own identity overshadowed, not because of how she presents herself, but because of how others view her, knowing she provides care:

> *The first question is always, "How's your mom?" It's never, "How are you, Kaci? What's going on? What's new in your life?" It's always, "How's your mom, tell me about your mom."*

The responsibility to family may also inhibit our participation in larger identity-building activities that unite others in our generation. One example became very apparent in 2020. Millennials are an activist generation;

when the Black Lives Matter protests were sweeping the country, we engaged deeply in the marches and in the conversation. But many caregivers couldn't join protests because of COVID precautions; preventing exposure of high-risk family was paramount. Caregivers were frustrated. Something big was happening in our society and they were lost as to how to take part. It spawned a discussion in Caregiver Collective of how people could participate, what they could do from home to still feel engaged and support the movement.

All this adds up to a particular breed of imposter syndrome, and caregivers our age "put on the mask" daily: we may present like we relate to our friends whose problems do not mirror our own…we belong to a generation whose representation doesn't always reflect us…we fake it till we make it with care responsibilities (which can even include medical tasks we convince ourselves we know how to do)…we front that we're able to nimbly balance providing care with everything else—because, really, we don't have a choice. But keeping quiet and pushing through only perpetuates the silence about Millennial caregivers and their disconnect from everyone else.

WHY IT'S IMPORTANT TO SELF-IDENTIFY

Lack of self-identification and awareness of others in the same boat prevent Millennial caregivers from knowing about and seeking available resources, from connecting with each other, and from just being real about who we are and how we're living. Just by identifying as a caregiver, here's what can change:

- Your self-esteem gets a boost, really. *The majority* of those who self-identified as caregivers believe their self-awareness led to increased confidence when talking to healthcare professionals about their loved one's care.[6] Knowing that you are the caregiver allows you to boss up, so to speak.
- You connect with the resources you need. *Over 90 percent* of family caregivers become more proactive about seeking out

needed resources and skills to assist their loved one after they have self-identified.[7]

- You connect with others you relate to, finally. Yes, I've shared how attending support groups led some caregivers our age to feel more ostracized, but the opposite effect can occur when you find the group right for you. I can't tell you how many people join Caregiver Collective and post something along the lines of *I'm so glad to find this group and meet others in the same boat as me* or introduce themselves by sharing *I haven't really told anyone I'm a caregiver*, and you can practically hear them sigh in relief to finally say it (or type it) out loud. Hearing from others dealing with similar situations, undergoing similar emotions you thought were yours to bear alone, can help to normalize this unique experience. You'll find you're in good company.

BALANCING YOUR IDENTITIES

Identity is about managing the various roles in our lives, even when family responsibilities feel all-consuming—*especially* when they do. It's critical for caregivers to define personal identities outside of caregiving or to get back in touch with their lives before. This is no easy task. It requires time and energy. But there's a reason those of us no longer in the caregiver role pass along the advice not to let your own life completely drop: because after caregiving, you'll need something to return to. And ultimately, you deserve to be *you*.

"Be specific about taking an inventory of your identity and really check in on what parts have taken a hit in caregiving and what you can do to preserve the other [parts]," advised Dr. Lisa Paz, a therapist experienced in counseling caregivers. "I'm picturing in my head a bar graph. Many different bars [make up your] identity.... When you're a student, a 'student' bar is much higher than (fill in the blank), the 'I like to exercise' or 'play music' bar. [The] caregiving bar becomes sort of the high bar, but it doesn't mean that the other features or metrics aren't in play." When thinking about the different "bars" that make up your identity, be careful not to overidentify with your caregiver role, even if it's the primary way you spend your time. "Take an assessment of how you want to be defined or what other parts of your identity maybe aren't going to hit the same height on the graph, but that still deserve either preservation or attention, and access it where you can."

This begs the question, How do I do this? I reached out to John Poole, who's been a member of Caregiver Collective from the beginning. When his parents both had strokes within a short time span, John gave up his career in politics and pursuit of his graduate degree to care for them full-time from home. Despite this massive commitment, John made time for some personal activities outside of care and, after both of his parents passed, he continues to provide guidance to other caregivers in the group about not giving up on themselves. I asked him how he did it and what advice he had:

> I was able to engage in activities for myself by enlisting the help of family and sometimes paid home health aides. I utilized their help if I wanted some downtime to go to the beach or see a stand-up comedy performance. I also think when caregivers are able to secure coverage for their loved ones, using it to go on a job interview or take a class would also be beneficial. I would also recommend not being shy about sharing some details of caregiving responsibilities with trusted friends. They may offer good advice.

What are the hobbies you love, the music you like to listen to, the foods you like to eat? These sound like small things, but caregivers might let them go. Instead, choosing them is choosing yourself and your Self. Incorporate them into your day or, if that's too high a bar, into your week.

How you convey your role to others, how you speak about yourself, is something to consider as well. We frequently hear people say, "I identify as ____," and then there's a whole news segment debating whether that identification is culturally permissible. Our question is, How do we label ourselves as caregivers in a way that is not so binary and doesn't preclude the other significant roles we inhabit?

I think it's important to think of ourselves as "caregiver and ____." When we share our career titles or our ethnic backgrounds, it informs the person with whom we're speaking about who we are, but they're aware that they're not getting the full picture from one statement; there are other aspects of who we are at play. We need to think of caregiving in the same way and not be afraid to share that role with people.

I'm a criminal defense attorney and the caregiver to my sister.

I'm a Black woman, climate activist, and caregiver to my dad.

I'm a registered voter, a mother, and a caregiver to my wife.

The way caregiving impacts our lives (such as through decreased wealth or status attainment, relationships, or family building) already influences other aspects of our identities and how we are viewed. We shouldn't shy away from who we are and how we spend our time. Caregivers are doing something incredibly worthwhile and impactful. Realize the value of who you are stating yourself to be.

RACIAL, ETHNIC, AND CULTURAL IDENTITIES SHAPE OUR CARE, TOO

Cultural identity and considerations factor into our care as well. Kaci told me how expectations instilled by her Polish heritage influence her ability to set caregiving boundaries and say no to her mom—in that it's pretty freaking difficult. "My mom was the first one born in this country in 1952. So having that immigrant background too, family is everything. It makes it very different."

Kaci is not the first caregiver I've spoken with who told me the family's cultural expectation of the younger caring for the elder gets translated into martyrdom, complete devotion with the loss of personal boundaries. She says when she talks to friends or colleagues who didn't have that type of upbringing, they don't understand why she doesn't just ignore her mom's phone call or go home later than she promised. (We'll get further into setting boundaries in a later chapter.) Maria, an expat friend of mine also of Polish descent, recently told me of the difficulties she's had arranging care for her mom, who lives in New Jersey and experiences mental health problems. Maria jumped through an extra hoop searching for a specialist who was not only appropriate for her mom's condition but also Polish-speaking and able to navigate her mom's cultural resistance to mental health treatment. There was also the job of convincing Maria's Polish father, who stigmatizes mental health issues and treatment and had her mom's ear.

Michelle told me that when it comes to her Asian American family, "There's just a lot of other considerations that are part of even reaching out for help" that are rooted in cultural norms and expectations. "I think it's been programmed in me for so long [not to ask relatives for help].... There's an Asian term about saving face, and there's just this sense of trying to always endure things and just put on a brave face and not really air dirty laundry out or ask for help or seem weak."

"In Asian communities it's a 'filial piety,' that sense of duty...specifically in their culture that they talk about. That is, this sense of honor that goes into multigenerational care," said Dr. Feylyn Lewis, a caregiving researcher. "I also think that that sense of duty and expectation and normalization of mutual care is a part of, I would say, Black and minority ethnic communities as well." Dr. Lewis, a Black American woman who was a youth caregiver to her mother, has written about the role of Black and African American culture as it relates to family care. In her experience, this expectation of multigenerational family care often falls to the women and girls of the family. "I'll speak for Black and those who identify as African Americans that, yeah, certainly, that is an expectation that women and girls are those who are best at care. They are more genetically suited to caregiving tasks. And of course we know that that is sexist." She laughed. "And, well, simply just false, because we know there's no special gene that we carry." That expectation of girls starts very young, she said.

As mentioned earlier, more than half of Millennial caregivers are people of color. It's important to recognize this diversity because of the economic repercussions caregiving has on our country's nonwhite populations. For example, Latinx Millennials face more intense pressure to balance care with employment than other Millennials do; they not only spend more time, on average, at work but also more frequently provide higher-hour levels of family care.[8] There are only so many hours in a day and, eventually, something may have to give. When a systemic issue like the accumulation of generational wealth is factored in, you can project how economic inequity may be exacerbated. Additionally, those younger Latinx caregivers born in the United States may feel torn between their culture's value of familism (the needs of the family being greater than the needs of the individual) and American assimilation.[9] According to the American Society on Aging, this may cause a rift between younger and older generations when priorities and expectations differ.

People of color have also reported "distinct care experiences and specific support needs" that require additional consideration (such as help with translation in doctor offices or other medical environments and specialized medical diets that take culture and tradition into account).[10] I've seen these cultural considerations also appear in different ethnic groups, like Kaci's Polish family.

THE INTERSECTION OF GENDER AND CAREGIVING

Despite expectations within the Black and African American community for women and girls to provide care, our generation's almost equal gender divide of caregivers was evident within Feylyn's own family: she was a youth caregiver, but it was her brother who dropped out of college to take over their mother's care in young adulthood. She had this observation:

Boys and men are hidden in our country as caregivers, they're not seen as much. Women and girls are the face of caregiving. I also feel it damages and harms them [men] as well. Because this myth that only girls and women can do caregiving or are good at caregiving…invalidates their experience and their competency, and quite frankly that's harmful. And of course, we know it's very damaging to maintain…and sustain sexist ideals for girls and women….

Even in my own family, I had intimately close family members say during the pandemic with my mother's stroke, "Oh, we're so glad that you're here to take care of your mom because your brother has work" and "Oh, there's nothing like daughters, you are the one to do the care." And it was very much understood that although my brother has been doing this for decades that, just because of my gender, I'm the better caregiver and the one that should be caregiving.

Feylyn found it "very funny" that her brother's career was prioritized while the two full-time jobs she was working were overlooked.

Brandon, who cares for his mom with Parkinson's, noticed that people treat him differently as a male caregiver in ways that, he says, make him feel guilty. "I feel like I get more praise and credit being a guy taking care of his mom, and then I'll feel guilty because it's like, well, I'm not doing anything more than countless women in these [caregiver support] groups with me, but it gets a little bit more attention." He says that although some people view his caregiving as "wholesome" and "cute," others, he believes, look at him with suspicion: unused to seeing men care for their moms, they might assume he's taking advantage of her in some way. At least they are looking out for her, he thinks.

Gendered stereotypes of care may screw with identity shaping for men in this role and can have a ripple effect of repercussions. "What we often see is it may increase some of those feelings of isolation," said Christina Irving, a licensed social worker and director of client services at Family Caregiver Alliance in San Francisco. "Because as hard as it can be for younger caregivers in general to feel like they have peers who are in that same space and going through the same thing, I think for male caregivers, because it doesn't fit that picture at any age as often, it may be harder to feel like there is that peer group in that same way, define that sense of identity."

Irving mentioned that gender norms also impact men in the role seeking help; they may face internal barriers in expressing emotion or admitting they can't do it all themselves. "It might be harder for younger male caregivers to talk about the emotional struggles both for and of their roles." Because their experience is not visibly normalized, it may feel challenging to find a support network of peers, but these connections can help men in the caregiver role find others modeling their experience, which can help them open up in ways that are more difficult to do with friends who don't understand the experience. "To have that space with people who are going through it, I think it gives permission and a sense of safety to them to feel like, 'Oh, I can say these things to him, I can bring up these issues and these challenges.'...I think the hardest part then is breaking through that initial barrier of events seeking out other caregivers." Caregiving support groups for men have become increasingly available, so consider this your informational kick in the butt to reach out.

Irving also says, "I think the more as a society we can normalize caregiving, and really how universal that experience is and normalize connecting with others, I think it then helps that individual caregiver be able to get past some of those internal or societal expectations and barriers." This normalization, I believe, would benefit us all.

PART TWO

FAMILY AND RELATIONSHIPS

CHAPTER 3

WHO WE CARE FOR

I WAS FOURTEEN WHEN THE MOVIE *CLUELESS* CAME OUT AND SOAKED US in a new vision for youth culture. Over a soundtrack boasting "we're the kids in America," we met blonde teen protagonist Cher: beautiful, confident, an only child whose mother died during routine surgery and whose father is a candidate for an imminent heart attack. Within the first minute of the movie, Cher lectures her dad on taking vitamins and drinking juice, reminds him about an upcoming doctor's appointment for his flu shot. Cher is coming of age, a kid in grown-up clothes, and assumed the role handed to her: woman of the house, concerned with her dad's health while also weighing her virginity and unable to pass her rite of passage road test. *Clueless* is a Beverly Hills–fueled satire, yes, but it models more about being a kid in America than I realized.

Even as a capable adult, around your parents you can assert authority but still feel so *young*. Taking charge of my dad's health introduced a role reversal that was difficult to admit. I was thirty-two when his condition worsened and daily needs related to his illness intensified. I wasn't married and didn't have kids of my own; my parents were the center of my family unit. At that age, I still leaned on them heavily, not for instruction but for guidance and wise companionship. I'd never been totally responsible for anyone but myself. His illness was the first real time my father depended on me and was vulnerable, and I assumed the responsibility with my heart and prioritized it. I always considered my dad before making my own plans. I paid his bills and helped him cut his food at meals. I made decisions on his behalf, like the nursing home he'd move into without him seeing it first, and with each decision I worried my choice was wrong, which meant something would go wrong. I felt the need to be his vocal cheerleader, advocate, strength and conditioning coach. I'd count off reps or miles when he was exercising in the physical therapy gym, encouraging him in a confident tone to push a little more but dropping the issue on days I sensed exhaustion.

The most significant role reversal was in who was providing who with strength. My dad was my vigilant protector, sheltering me in the comfort of safety and the knowledge everything would be alright; now I was needed to show him reassurance, to project a well of confidence he could draw from. When I was a preteen, my dad once told me, "One day you'll realize your parents are just people." He meant that they, too, are fallible; they make mistakes despite best intentions. Watching him push against physical limitations of his mortality, I saw a different version. I didn't see him as "just" a person, but in some moments I glimpsed a mortal man who could be scared, lack defenses that I had been accustomed to protecting both of us for decades. Seeing the "strong" one expose vulnerability was like a quick knife in the heart; he was human.

As my dad's dependence on me grew, I restrained my reliance on him. Speaking became increasingly difficult for him, so I was conscientious about which questions I'd ask that sought full thoughts beyond straightforward one-word answers. To fully vocalize required increasing effort, it took time, and in response the number of topics we covered in a single conversation became fewer. I could carry conversation like a monologue he engaged with, took pleasure and entertainment from, but the deeper questions I limited to what I needed his feedback on most; the issues, real or just swirling in my head, that I knew he'd enjoy ruminating and giving thoughts on, the stuff I really needed my dad for. It was painful to ignore the other questions—Should I move neighborhoods? Take the job that feels like a professional compromise?—when all I wanted was my father's reassuring voice and familiar advice, solicited or not. He had a very particular point of view with a disregard for outside judgment, which often boiled down to "fuck 'em." He could see my problems simply while I spiraled with possible versions, and the plainness removed some of the weight.

Meanwhile, trying to assert any authority over the man I once helplessly called from three thousand miles away with a flat tire was like a joke to both of us. Any stern instruction I tried to give, about practicing voice exercises or strengthening his neck muscles, were totally undermined and came across as more nuisance than wisdom. It didn't help that my skills navigating his wheelchair were downright dangerous. I regularly smashed the side of his chair, with accompanying fingers or arms, into doorframes. If a sidewalk sloped, I'd grip the rubber handles tighter, throw my full body weight back, and pray he wouldn't fly out of the seat as I tried to veer back on course. He found my haplessness funny and would laugh to the point of crying; despite being a grown woman he marveled at, I was still his little girl and a bit of a mess. I think, for him, it made everything feel more normal. I was a Daddy's Girl in a woman's body. The adult responsibility I took for him couldn't have been heavier, and I was capable, but at times it was comforting to loosen my grip on maturity, just a bit.

Caring for parents—or grandparents—is the most common care relationship of our generation (sometimes it's even both at once), but it's far from the only one.[1] When examined in totality, *who* Millennials are caring for may have surprised you before you began reading: yes, some of us aid these senior family members, but an incredible number of us care for spouses and partners. We also care for siblings and chosen family (like friends and neighbors).

No matter the relationship, as caregiving duties evolve and expand, these relationships change in ways that feel unexpected when they are, in fact, common. We may experience *role ambiguity*, a redefining of the relationship to the care recipient.[2] We grapple with reconciling who the person was, who they are, and who they will be along with who we are to them. I was always my father's daughter first, but his disease shifted our dynamic to incorporate my new responsibility. I never introduced myself as his caregiver, ever, but the definition of *daughter* and what I wanted it to convey when I met a doctor or called an insurance provider meant something new. (I'll give you an example. If I felt my dad was being shoved aside or wasn't receiving the medical attention he needed in that moment, I'd say, "I'm Jennifer, I'm his *daughter*," which meant: Do not fuck with me, I will throw fire to protect him.)

A friend recently told me that she was examining the support she gave her mom, who has mental illness, and was having a hard time differentiating which responsibilities she took on because she was her mom's daughter, her caregiver, or subconsciously "parenting" her mother. Experiencing this role ambiguity at a younger age, whether with a parent or spouse or any of these fluctuating care relationships, can create confusion and challenges.

Role ambiguity can also happen with other people in our life outside of caregiving but because of caregiving. Often, providing care for someone means our other care relationships—to our friends, other family members, and ourselves—get put on a back burner. A close friend may question whether they can still come to us for advice or support like they used to or whether their needs will fall on closed ears because we are overwhelmed with caregiving. When we refer to "who we care for," we need to remember caregiving doesn't happen in a vacuum and is a major role taken on in tandem with other relationships in our lives. (Multigenerational caregivers who provide care for an adult while also raising kids have acute insight into this—something we'll get deeper into later in this book.)

Let's dig into the most common caregiving scenarios for our youngish generation today.

PARENT

The parent-child role reversal that I experienced felt so personal but is a textbook repercussion of caring for a parent. I hear so many caregivers our age refer to it as "parenting their parent." Like me, many take on parental care before they've had kids of their own, so having a dependent is new, a role not already occupied by little ones—maybe for this reason the metaphor comes more easily. The tasks are out of our ordinary but undoubtedly similar to those of parents: you may be feeding, bathing, paying for, and assuming overall responsibility for the parent who once cared for you. They now have a dependence on you that is hard to deny. There also may be a lot of tying of shoes. Nevertheless, we need to be careful with the "parenting my parent" comparison.

When I saw that the first article I wrote about caring for my dad had been titled by the editor "I Became My Father's Parent at 32," I thought, *Oh no*. I didn't feel that way. Yes, I had assumed a new responsibility, but I was not my dad's parent: he was still the one who shepherded my values, advised me on right from wrong, protected me. He was not naive; he just needed help. What I was doing may have superficially looked similar to parenting, may have been an easy comparison to make to succinctly convey my responsibilities (especially for a curiosity-provoking headline), but was very different. The respect and deference I had for my dad had not changed. Some Millennial caregivers really take offense to this language, feeling it infantilizes their loved one—and I understand that; it implies a power dynamic that is unfair and can be seen as belittling.

Ultimately, caring for a parent at a young age, and the subsequent role reversal, can create a devastating *ambiguous loss*, or grief for the person they "were" and the role they played (or you hoped they would play) in your life. If you are younger and providing care, you may feel like you're growing up faster than your peers when you sense the lack of parental guidance; hell, even older Millennials can feel this way. Despite the parent physically being there, this perceived loss can affect the parent–adult child relationship in its current state. Take Michelle: she's been caring for her mom in some ways since she was a teenager; now, with Michelle in her early thirties, her mom's renal disease has progressed to a terminal stage and Michelle's caregiver duties have intensified. Her mom's changed physical state changed their relationship:

Before her condition escalated, I was pretty close with my mom.... Over time we're still good, but I think our relationship has evolved and a lot of

it has been as a result of becoming that caretaker role. In some ways, I do
feel myself distancing a little because the relationship is not as two-way as
it used to be. Whenever we are together, it's very heavy on the giving on
my part. I think I've sensed that over time we've become less close because
of that.

I've spoken with multiple caregivers who've said that so much of their time with their parent is taken up by care—making sure appointments are set, that the person has eaten, taken their medications (and are the meds working?)—that they feel there's little space or energy left for their actual interpersonal relationship. Conversation is dominated by care tasks, and they begin to think of their parent as a patient. The sense of loss is intensified. I refused to let go of my father as my parent and held on tight, prioritizing quality time and conversation; yes, the disease was always present, but it wasn't always focused on. We genuinely liked each other, so it's what we both wanted, whether it was stated or not, and felt most authentic. (We'll go deeper into various stages of grief in a later chapter.)

Adjusting to role reversal and role ambiguity is not something we undergo alone—our parents may go through it, too. Suddenly, kiddo's medical opinions and learned expertise are the predominant voice in the room, and that can take getting used to. Laura, a school friend of mine, told me that after her dad had surgery on his jaw, they butted heads discussing his further medical treatments: "It was late at night after surgery and he [was] kind of not wanting me to interfere. He didn't think I knew what I was doing."

Preexisting strains in your relationship can make the care scenario more uncomfortable or feel burdensome. In Caregiver Collective, I ended up forming a breakout group for the adult children of alcoholics who had now assumed care for their parent. They grappled with an entirely different set of emotional issues, particularly resentment of their parent, that they found common ground on and were able to support each other through. Another member took on care for her estranged father who, she says, she had never forgiven for abusing her mother; still, she couldn't leave him by the wayside. In these cases, the "quality time" ideal doesn't have the same meaning as it did for me or for Laura.

Even when relationships aren't strained, they can be difficult. Before COVID, Ron had taken steps to move his mother, who has experienced mental illness for most of Ron's life, into her own apartment with hired aides so that he could attain some breathing room that he hadn't had for much his adulthood. Ron told me how the pandemic, particularly cohabitating again during lockdown, reignited parent-child issues from earlier in life:

> *That's someone you love and want to be close to, but as you "adult" and individuate you also need separation from. It was a very confusing time because I had fought so much for that individuation and separation. I put so much effort and work into doing that, just both for myself and especially in a caregiving situation. It's different when you're individuating from a parent [while] growing up, but then it's hard to individuate from a parent that really can't function without your support.*

PARTNER OR SPOUSE

The age of people who provide care for a spouse or partner is also getting younger. Two major events influenced how many of us are already caring for a romantic partner: 9/11 and the COVID pandemic.

Post-9/11 alone, over a million military caregivers were added—most under the age of thirty.[3] Eldest Millennials were twenty at the time of 9/11, so we are in the crosshairs of this stat. Caregivers for these veterans who served in the wake of September 11 (often spouses) tend to be caring for someone with a mental health or substance abuse issue. The veteran caregivers I've spoken to were often caring for someone with traumatic brain injury in addition to other physical impairments. Beth was one of the first Millennial caregivers I connected with when I created the Collective. At the time, Beth was in her twenties and had been caring for her veteran husband for a few years, since he'd been injured by an improvised explosive device (IED). To help with his care, she had to drop out of graduate school and work multiple jobs, and she was fired from one company when he was hospitalized for an extended period.

Think tank RAND Corporation noted this group of younger veteran caregivers needs long-term support because their age may make the future of their current support systems uncertain, as they may be in new marriages or rely heavily on aging parents.[4]

In 2020, AARP released a report that stated 20 percent of all caregivers between the ages of eighteen and forty-nine were caring for a spouse or partner.[5] The report explicitly stated research was conducted prior to the pandemic. It's important to account for COVID when considering how many of us are caring for partners today. I think it's a valid assumption that the number is higher than 20 percent in the pandemic's wake. The Centers for Disease Control and Prevention (CDC) reported that the prevalence of long COVID in the United States is highest among those between the ages of thirty-five and forty-four, aimed squarely at our generation.[6] Although still an illness that is not completely understood, the symptoms of long COVID can be debilitating (including extreme fatigue, sensitivity to touch or sound, depression, and brain fog).[7] As of now, there is no known treatment or cure; home care, or at least assistance, is often required for these Millennials with long COVID. The spousal caregivers interviewed for this book coincidentally had partners diagnosed with long COVID or a similar undiagnosed affliction contracted during the pandemic. These caregivers are unsure whether their partners will require care for another year or forever.

Lizzie, a thirty-four-year-old mom who cares for her husband with long COVID, is emblematic of how the classic sandwich generation has evolved for our generation into the multigenerational caregiver—caring for multiple family members of, you guessed it, different generations; in Lizzie's case, her husband and children. Since COVID, in particular, the age of multigenerational caregivers has become younger as more of us take on care of an affected spouse (or sibling).[8]

When her husband contracted long COVID, Lizzie's world was turned upside down and hasn't recovered. She wrestles with the idea of considering herself a single parent to their two small children, but that's how she feels. While he is on medical leave from his job, Lizzie has continued working while raising their kids; because her husband has a hard time focusing, is unable to read, and has extreme fatigue, she has taken the reins on his medical care and treatment. She keeps a binder to catalog his symptoms, treatments they've attempted, and the results. After months of trying, he was finally accepted to one of the few long COVID treatment programs in the country. Even with this large hurdle accomplished, Lizzie is daunted by the prospect that his illness, and their current family situation, is indefinite. She told me that she only allows herself to plan ahead one year at a time, mostly to make sure that childcare is covered for any upcoming work trips or weddings.

Her reluctance to think too far into the future is understandable: there are major financial and emotional implications for members of our generation providing care for decades. Not only is more out-of-pocket cash going toward the person's care for longer, but Lizzie also has to contend with the cost of childcare: with her husband no longer able to share kid-watching duties, Lizzie needs someone from the outside to help, and family isn't always available. Your partner's income contribution or health benefits may also be in jeopardy if they are no longer employed full-time or at all. The added pressure around money creates additional stress for a young (or younger) partnership that is already dealing with a lot.

SIBLINGS

Some of us are caregivers to siblings who are unable to hold steady employment or to care for themselves because of a chronic condition.[9] Like caregiving for a romantic partner or friend, this role may last your entire lifetime. The support given can come in the form of "typical" care responsibilities, such as assisting someone who is physically disabled, or financial support. Those who began caring for a sibling from a young age (possibly childhood) may mature at a faster rate than they otherwise would have, as they assume substantial responsibilities like wheelchair transfers or medication management early in life. There are cases where the caregiving sibling may feel like they are being taken advantage of and will never lead a life independent of their sibling; the care recipient may feel resentful of being dependent and not "in control." These can add an intense layer to "typical" sibling rivalry. Even when feelings of resentment are not an issue, the caregiving sibling may become preoccupied with figuring out things to improve their sibling's quality of life, like activities or hobbies they can manage, or can feel pressure to plan and "live life" for both of them.

Those who begin caring in adulthood may have to assume their sibling's life roles and responsibilities in addition to providing care. Katie took in her sister, who had terminal cancer, and her sister's two children. In her early forties and married with kids of her own, Katie struggled to manage all the family demands with her own career and hospice care for her sister. She expressed pain watching her sister suffer but also grappled with figuring out how to comfort her sister's kids in the process of losing their mom.

NON-BIO "CHOSEN" FAMILY MEMBERS

Historically, we've heard about "chosen" family usually in the context of the LGBTQ+ community, in cases when people estranged from their biological family—because of gender identity or sexual orientation—create surrogate family units with friends. (The forming of these chosen families was particularly big at the height of the AIDS epidemic in the 1980s.) Although this type of family formation still occurs today, I've also observed chosen families born for a variety of other reasons, particularly when caregiving is required. People may assume care for their widowed older neighbor who has no living family but continues living at home, the "uncle" you're not actually related to, the stepmom who is no longer married to your dad and who doesn't have biological children, a friend whose family can't—or won't—offer the care they need.

Mia, who cares for her best friend, a veteran with severe injuries, said his family is in the picture but in denial about the severity of his condition; she's witnessed incidents when they've interfered with his treatment and believes they don't take his medical needs seriously. She undertakes his care on her own, feeling it's her responsibility.

In 2015, 16 percent of Millennial caregivers were caring for a friend or neighbor.[10] Though research is sparse, I have to guess that this number has increased in the wake of long COVID as our generation is sitting at the crossroads of high prevalence of the disease and low marriage rates. Although chosen family caregivers critically fill a void in care, they are often not legally recognized as family—which, when it comes to dealing with hospitals or employers, is severely problematic.

WHEN THE GOVERNMENT DEFINES WHO YOUR FAMILY IS

As of now, the relationships considered "family" under various laws and government protections, such as family leave benefits, are either set at the state level or dictated by the federal Family and Medical Leave Act (FMLA). These laws are specific about who is eligible to receive benefits and what their legal relationship to the care recipient is. For example, a sister in New Jersey can legally take time off work to care for her brother with cancer, but an adult sister in Ohio is at risk of being terminated from her job for doing the same thing. (By the way, honorable mention to the state of New Jersey, which legally acknowledges caregiving for families of all types, including chosen family.) FMLA (if applicable) limits qualifications for caring to a child, spouse, parent, or parental figure.[11]

In medical environments, we often hear about this as an issue in the case of couples who are not legally married, whether LGBTQ+ or heteronormative; some laws prohibit an unmarried partner from visiting the other in the hospital, having access to their medical information, or making critical medical decisions in case of an emergency. Although the person requiring care considers their partner to be family, the law might not. This could leave the person requiring care at the decision-making mercy of family unfamiliar with their wishes or unwilling to abide by them—or with no one, legally, to act on their behalf. In caregiving, this discrimination also occurs in biological families when the relationship is not considered "family enough" to be a caregiver (such as the earlier example of siblings). It's a system at odds with how care looks in our country; it's a system at odds with family as our generation (and generations before and after us) defines it. If our medical system is leaning on adults of all ages to provide family care, then our laws need to include and protect those same adults when it comes to caregiver rights.

CHAPTER 4

WHERE WE LIVE AND WHO WE LIVE WITH

IN MY LATE TWENTIES AND EARLY THIRTIES, I WAS LIVING ACROSS THE country from my dad, who was in assisted living. After a bad fall and subsequent time spent in in-patient rehab, we learned my father was not allowed to return to his assisted living apartment: the plastic brace-let that marked him as a "fall risk" branded him unsafe if unsupervised; his building's regulations demanded a higher level of care that required he move into a nursing home. The decision of where needed to be made immediately. I flew home at once to tour nursing homes with my mom. I didn't tell anyone where I was off to; I think my coworkers assumed I was off partying. I loudly questioned the bureaucratic decision that made this move necessary, worried it would set my dad back further. Quietly, I wondered what this change indicated about the true state of his health. My mother repeated that she felt terrible he could not return to what had become his home.

Assisted living had been great. My dad had a private studio apartment filled with his own furniture and belongings. The bathroom was large enough to accommodate a wheelchair, which he didn't need then, and felt spacious by New York City standards. There he had hung a framed painting I did as a child—in my dad's opinion, your favorite artwork was hung in the bathroom where you could contemplate it quietly and alone. Assisted living organized his doctor appointments and transportation, they managed his medications, he could come and go independently, but his exits and presence for meals in the dining room were monitored. He, we, had assembled a friend community in place there. In many ways it was a relief, we *liked it*, so it was a blow to be told he had to leave. In its place was the heavy decision I'd need to make on my dad's behalf while under a ticking clock.

The first nursing home my mom and I entered, I burst into tears. It felt cold, institutional. *Was this how they would all be? Is this just something to accept, that I'm sending my dad to live in a place I want to run right out of?* I had to get through this. Waiting at the elevator, I put on my sunglasses. I told myself to look for silver linings, quality of care. We entered the cafeteria and it was a horror: people, some still in pajamas, left in their chairs alone in the room, no interaction, no visible care. Well after mealtime, they were just *there*. I wondered if they had families. I couldn't believe anyone would allow a loved one to live in such a place. It cemented that I would advocate closely and fiercely for my dad; I would need to.

One of the next places was *bouj*, a bit far but on beautiful grounds, known for its world-class art collection. I arrived with hope. When we met for the tour, one of the first questions an administrator asked was how we would pay for it. Although I'm sure the care they provide is good, this encounter left me with the impression that their priorities didn't align with what we were seeking.

Another home we toured was one my mom was familiar with and had great amenities—including a pub. Residents sipped beers while watching that afternoon's game on TV; it was clearly social and across the street from a renowned hospital. The décor was nice but stuffy, old New York leather and wood paneling. When I was a kid, my dad owned a modern art gallery, and he had a previous career as an interior designer. Style wasn't our top priority, but if we could, we wanted to make sure he had the sense he was "home." As we went from home to home, my mom and I kept my dad informed on where we were looking; he quietly thumbed through brochures while we told him our thoughts. We wanted him to feel involved, agency at a time the torch of decision-making had silently been passed.

My mom and I traveled uptown to a beautiful neighborhood by Columbia University. It was quieter than downtown but buzzed with university students and families. This home was across the street from St. John the Divine (one of the most beautiful cathedrals in New York) and a large park, it shared the neighborhood with good restaurants and bookstores. A bakery both my parents knew from life before me was down the block. There was an excellent hospital across the street. Walking in, I felt cheerful: the furniture and wallpaper weren't super fancy but well-kept and comfortable. There was action, activities going on on each floor, regular musical performances and ice cream socials on the calendar, daily physical therapy not only offered but encouraged; they made sure every resident got dressed in the morning. Lining the length of the building was a patio overlooking the sidewalk, where we could push my dad's chair to sit outside on nice afternoons, to eat at one of the umbrellaed tables or to people watch. In the summers, they hosted barbecue lunches there. This would be it; it needed to be.

(I'd like to note that I've spoken to caregivers across the country, so I realize one reaction to this may be: *Sure you had nice choices, but they all require a ton of money we don't have.* To dispel this assumption, our list consisted of only the homes my dad's insurance fully covered. Beds for his insurance may have been limited, maybe there was a waitlist, but we were willing to get resourceful to get one. The biggest advantage we had, I see clearly now in retrospect, was our location: New York City offers access to some amazing resources, whereas not everyone's location offers the same.)

The nursing home provided a wholesome world-within-a-world. Some of the people working there were so dedicated to brightening the lives of residents—planning activities, always smiling and chatting in the elevator, laughing about how my father was the ladies' man of the building—that they shone from within and spread that light. Watching them, I had the genuine feeling that these humans were somehow angels on earth. Something about the nursing home felt so safe and contained, the world outside less secure in comparison. It was a strange dichotomy, spending afternoons there at oldies singalongs, then leaving to meet friends and strangers in loud, dark bars that night.

When my dad moved into the nursing home, it wasn't just a location change; the power dynamic between us shifted with responsibilities redistributed. Deciding where our family member lives when they are in need of care is a consideration we all face, whether preemptively or in the heat of urgency. What we don't discuss is how *where* they live affects *how* we live, too, and our generation's profile plays a role.

IT'S TRUE, MORE MILLENNIALS LIVE WITH THEIR PARENTS—HERE'S WHY

During the initial pandemic lockdowns, maybe you noticed a phenomenon of Millennial and Gen Z adults cohabitating with older relatives. New York's then-Governor Andrew Cuomo's infamous daily addresses often included anecdotes about living with his three twenty-something daughters, all of whom moved home to lock down with him. It was a window into what was going on nationally: over half of all eighteen- to twenty-nine-year-olds began living with parents during that first phase of the pandemic, surpassing the previous peak during the Great Depression.[1] This trend existed for men and women, across all major racial and ethnic groups, in both metropolitan areas and rural, in all four main Census regions of the United States. By April 2020, more than thirty-two million adults lived with a parent or grandparent, a 10 percent spike from a year earlier.[2] (A large majority of these adults were Gen Z in part because of college closures.) A drop in the employment rate of young adults during this time was partially to blame, but this intense period was reflective of a larger movement in the United States that had begun pre-COVID.

"Millennials have led the movement toward multigenerational households," wrote *USA Today* in 2020, citing Census info from 2015. In 2018, sixty-four million Americans were living in multigenerational households—the highest number on record and an increase of almost 70 percent from 1980, when the eldest Millennials were busy being conceived.[3] Prepandemic, 15 percent of Millennials were living in their parents' home, a higher proportion than Gen X and nearly double the rate of Boomers at the same age.[4] Education played a role: those who never attended college were twice as likely to live at home than those Millennials who held a bachelor's degree or higher. When Gen Z is taken into account, almost half of employed young adults lived in a parent's home.[5] It's important we understand *why*.

The "lazy Millennials living in Mom's basement" trope was fatally punctured during the pandemic news cycle, when mass media finally acknowledged the economic turbulence Millennials have been wrapped up in since the eldest of us graduated from college (if the threat of lifetime student loan repayments didn't hold us back from attending). Intergenerational households often reflect this financial insecurity: Some Millennials live with parents until they have stable salaries and can afford their own place. Others choose to cohabitate with parents once they have kids (retired parents provide free live-in childcare). Boomers, generally, are not as well off as their own parents were—in part because they are retiring at the same age but living much longer. They may feel an economic squeeze, too, with their kids left to cover costs, which can mean taking in parents. Other reasons are cultural, based on our generation's diverse racial and ethnic backgrounds in which adult children cohabitate with one or both parents even later in life; 29 percent of people from Asian descent in the United States live in multigenerational households, for example (compared with 16 percent of white Americans).[6] Because future generations of Americans are projected to be more diverse than those of today, we should consider multigenerational households a fixture.[7] Another big reason our generation chooses multigenerational households: some people just *like it*; they're close to their parents or grandparents and want to raise their own kids within a close family unit.

Though Millennials are shifting family dynamics under a single roof, there is still stigma attached to multigenerational households, as if cohabitating is a signal of "failure to launch." I recently listened to an episode of The Cut's podcast that highlighted employed, accomplished youngish adults who made this choice willingly, happily, but still didn't admit their living situations to peers or coworkers for fear of judgment. When we hear about someone living with their family, rather than rush to judgment we should understand the gamut of reasons that may have led to the decision and accept that it's pretty common. Understanding the reasons our generation leads the trend toward multigenerational households also informs why so many of us cohabitate with the person we care for.

CAREGIVING UNDER THE SAME ROOF

Among Millennials, living with the person you care for in order to manage their care appears to be the most predominant situation. For many of them, this choice to share a home often doesn't *feel* like a choice at all. Many reluctantly moved back home (or never left) to prevent a loved one from moving into a living facility, or they installed a wheelchair ramp and hospital-grade bed into the new home they had hoped to share with a future partner. When you are younger, especially if you are unmarried, it can be viewed as most feasible for you to uproot your life and move in with your parent—or, depending on how early you began caregiving, never move out at all.

Some caregivers live with their parents because they cannot fathom how to pay for the long-term care their loved one needs, whether round-the-clock aides or a viable live-in care facility. They *would* choose a good nursing home if, financially, it was an option. The cost of live-in facilities, like assisted living or a nursing home, is exorbitant in the United States if you don't have long-term care insurance or low-income Medicaid benefits. Other people won't consider the idea of a live-in facility, or they prefer to care for their family at home.

COVID quickly made the living-together scenario far more likely: for caregivers who lived apart from their relative, the inability to find safe in-home or day care forced their choice to be under the same roof. "The pandemic is reshaping the way Americans care for the elderly, prompting family decisions to avoid nursing homes and keep loved ones in their own homes for rehabilitation and other care," wrote the *Wall Street Journal* in December 2020. By then more than 115,000 COVID deaths were linked to long-term care facilities and, if they could, families were moving their loved ones *out*. It set off a significant decline in nursing home admissions, a trend that looks to be continuing and that will increase the likelihood of home sharing.[8] Coupled with nursing home labor shortages and chronic government underfunding, nursing homes have been forced to decrease admissions or even shut down entirely.[9] It's led to a growing national crisis in access to nursing home care, further limiting it as a housing option.

The choice (or lack of choice) to live together can be accompanied, depending on our age and life stage, by a sense that the dreams we have for ourselves as young adults are dashed. Our generation is more likely to seek work abroad, and caregiving may put those dreams on hold indefinitely.[10] Some just wanted to attend college out of state but felt they needed to stay home and instead chose a school in their hometown. When we're sharing a home, both dating and personal boundaries feel impossible. But still, we commit to these living arrangements, and more often than previous generations have.

MICHELLE STAYED AT HOME

Michelle, whose mom has renal disease, lived in her parents' home for thirty years. Caregiving played a role in where she lived her entire adult life. She says she began caregiving for her mom when she was about fifteen or sixteen years old but didn't consider herself a caregiver until reflecting on it as an adult: "When it became [that] it wasn't just like you're hanging out with your mom, it's like you're going out with your mom because she needs stability to stand up straight because she might fall." A native New Yorker, Michelle chose to attend college in the city and moved into dorms farther uptown. After graduation she moved back in with her parents, mostly to get her footing. She was present to help her mom on "off" days but wasn't really needed at home...until, over time, the "off" days became more frequent. Helping at home went from being a convenience that Michelle could accommodate to a necessity: it

became evident her mom's capabilities were deteriorating and that someone needed to be with her at all times. What started out as being an extra
set of hands became helping her mom with daily meal prep, which progressed to taking over cooking; the kitchen was reflective of the larger
responsibility Michelle had assumed.

She had never intended to live at home forever. "There were moments
when I thought of moving out, and then it was like, but what would we
do? And then it's like, that thought process sort of ended." Her desire
for independence, to live in her own place, was stifled not just by being
needed at home but also by everything that came with living with your
parents and living in service of someone who needs help. Michelle used
her job as a strategist for a design firm as an outlet for freedom, an environment where she could be herself and express her independence and
work toward her goals. Michelle felt like an outlier among peers, living
with her parents to provide her mom's care, but her situation is quite
common: of the millions of Millennials already caring for a parent, over
60 percent are living in the parents' home.[11]

In 2019, Michelle's mom's health hit relative stability; overall, the family was managing life with chronic disease. With things at home steady,
Michelle turned her attention to a major work opportunity: she had started
in a two-year program at her company, at the end of which it was her goal
to relocate to a different office in another country. This had been her intention since the beginning and now it was in her sights. For Michelle, the
potential for this meant so much:

> For me, this was going to be a really big exciting thing that I was going to
> undertake. And also one of the first times that I would do something for
> me…doing something that puts me first and what I wanted to do and what
> my goals were versus, "Oh, it would be helpful to be at home and help out
> more." So I started telling people, "Okay, I'm gonna make this happen. I'm
> gonna relocate to our company's Singapore office." It was gonna be a really
> great experience not only relocating but also going to a different country to
> live for the first time and live on my own for the first time since undergrad.

Michelle met with the Singapore office leadership and received an offer. Ecstatic, she went home—but before she could share the news, her mom informed her that she'd seen her doctor: she was in end-stage renal disease. Michelle didn't tell her parents about the offer; instead, she emailed office leadership, telling them thanks, but a family matter had come up.

Michelle told me she could have gone anyway; chronic illness persists over time; her mom wouldn't decline drastically tomorrow. The choice to stay, she says, was hers. I asked her why she made that decision. "A sense of family obligation. And I think also fear of what could happen if you shirk that obligation."

Michelle continued living at home, managing the household, operating her mom's daily dialysis treatments, and sleeping in her childhood bedroom... which also became her home office during the pandemic. Her parents took her 24/7 presence as a sign she was available to help them at any time; they would pop into her room while she was on Zoom meetings; her dad would wake her from sleep to help out with something. Whereas before Michelle used working as an escape for her sense of self, she now used it as an excuse to just physically be in a separate room. It was during that time of nonstop living, working, and caregiving at home that Michelle hit a big breaking point:

> It was being at home all the time, even on the off hours or on the weekends.... You don't have your escape activities. You don't have your self-care activities, or whatever, outside. And then again, you're in this environment that reiterates that your needs aren't really the priority. And so that on its own can get really overwhelming. And then the other part of it is just the grief of it, of the sickness. So what I would do is hunker down in my room.
>
> I just got to a point, another breaking point. I was like, I need to get out. I need to change my environment. And I need to do it safely.

Apartment hunting in 2020 felt too risky for her, health-wise; she had to remain conscientious about the virus to protect her parents, especially her mom. Instead, she began to look for an Airbnb around November 2020; in April 2021, one year into the pandemic, she booked a short-term rental to stay for a period of three months. She made sure the apartment was within walking distance so she could still help at home; she just needed to tell her parents. The conversation did not go smoothly. Her parents brought up reasons and excuses for her not to leave. "They weren't fully getting why I needed it," Michelle said. "And to be fair, I don't think I ever fully expressed the toll of caretaking to them because I also don't feel like I can or that it would help anything. Or I feel like it would just make them feel worse. But I think ultimately what ended up happening was, I was like, 'It's not something I want. It's something that I need right now.' [I] just needed my own space to figure out what I want and like to do."

Michelle moved into the Airbnb, a huge step for her independence, but the reprieve didn't last long. Her mom had a fall and Michelle was needed at home again, at least for a bit. Afterward, she still had about a month of her contract remaining to peacefully live in her own space; in that time, she was able to contrast the environment she had always lived in, been accustomed to, with what it was like to really be on her own in a place where she called the shots.

It turned out what she wanted to do was spend time quietly being creative. She picked up a sketchpad, resumed hobbies and interests she had put aside because she hadn't had time. They were small interests that she didn't know she still had.

"I feel like a kid and an adult all in one. I kind of joke, it's like I skipped childhood and then I went straight into being a parent with the role reversal in a way. And I felt like there's some place in the middle where I just didn't fully experience that, that part of life."

RON STAYED CLOSE

For Ron, caregiving also always influenced where he lived and went to school. When he was younger, Ron and his family lived in Miami. His father died when Ron was fourteen, and by the time he was sixteen, his mother began displaying signs of psychiatric mental illness, something Ron thinks was present long before but that his father had shielded him and his sister from. In high school, Ron already felt the need to financially provide and logistically support his mom. When it came time for college, despite looking at schools in California and Washington, DC, Ron remained in Miami.

Ron did move to New York City for law school; his mom stayed in Miami, where his sister was able to be present for her. She and their mom don't share the same relationship as Ron does, he said, so he was still caregiving for his mother long distance and traveling to Miami every two weeks. "A big part of what I was doing while I was getting my education is constantly, even when it was from afar, constantly going back and forth and trying to make sure that there was…food and shelter for this person who was not well.…It wasn't a good situation for many years." For a time, his mother traveled between Miami and Ron's New York apartment, but it wasn't sustainable. Eventually, he moved her in with him.

When I first met Ron through the caregiver group years ago, he and his mom were living together in Manhattan. I remember him talking about needing to leave the office and skip after-work networking to get home to her; she had psychotic episodes and someone needed to be around to ground her back into reality, to combat voices she might have been hearing. Ron's life revolved around his mom's care and his high-intensity career in finance; the pressure to provide was tremendous, and he needed space of his own. For a while, he considered moving his mom into her own apartment and hiring aides to supervise her but didn't know whether it was feasible. Eventually, Ron moved his mom into her own place not far away in Queens while he remained in Manhattan:

> To be transparent, that's a big part of the roller coaster of caregiving because, technically, it's a huge expense for me. I'm not independently wealthy. I work for every penny, I put myself through school.…Now that I'm having to use my earnings that I work so hard for to keep two apartments, and then the

only reason I have a second one is for her to live in and to care for her, brings up a lot of [emotional] noise. It would for anyone.

Let me reiterate: Ron is paying two New York City rents. Aside from the financial burden, it seemed to be working for him...until the pandemic lockdowns. Then, as many caregivers experienced, home health aides were not able to continue working. Ron, again, took up the mantle—both living with his mom and caring for her—while working remotely from her home. He said that during that intense period he neglected himself and his own needs. Eventually, as things reopened, he was able to return to life in his own place—but it's never full-time. He describes his life now as "nomadic." Depending on his mom's condition any given day, Ron will stay with her and spend the night. When she's mentally stable again, he'll commute back to his place for a night or three:

The wear and tear on my body constantly going back and forth, it's just a constant. Sometimes I'm back and forth twice in a day....

There's a lot that you're doing logistically, mentally, not having a routine for yourself. So I think on the surface it can sound like a really good setup, and then when you start to dig into it, it's a sacrifice I'm making for my sanity. Absolutely. And I question whether it's the right sacrifice or not.

CASEY MOVED IN

Casey lives with the person she cares for, but the situation is different entirely: he's now her husband. Casey is a thirty-five-year-old graphic designer living in New Mexico. When we first spoke, she was two years into caregiving for her forty-two-year-old then-boyfriend whose debilitating chronic illness began during the pandemic. It remains undiagnosed but presents similarly to chronic fatigue syndrome. "One day [he] was feeling a little bit sick and within four days, he was just completely unrecognizable. He could barely walk. He could barely talk. We went to the emergency room several times. Nobody knew what was wrong." It was his need for in-home care that informed when and how they began living together and to such a degree that it's had a significant impact on her life and their relationship. In particular, their families did not understand or support them moving in together, despite his illness.

Their traditional religious upbringings precluded living together before marriage; but traditional ideals didn't account for the illness he contracted during lockdown. At the time, Casey lived in her own Albuquerque apartment about five minutes away from her boyfriend's house. After a second ER trip in two weeks, she decided to stay in his guest room so that if he needed something but couldn't get to a phone, he could just knock on the wall.

Cohabitating became more permanent when her lease ran out and, caregiving still needed, she moved into his guest room full-time. Her belongings in storage, she told me that even eight months in she felt somewhat homeless. "It's just super weird to kind of give up your whole life and your identity." Each time she referred to her home, I noticed, she referred to it as "his place."

"I just feel like I live here. We don't share finances. We are our own separate people living under the same roof for medical reasons, so part of my brain just is not going to accept that this place is mine until there's a marriage license." There's a possibility that you're reading this thinking the arrangement was a convenient ploy for two religious people to live together before marriage, or that it's an argument to rush a wedding. But Casey's home life is not what you'd imagine for two carefree young adults setting up house. Because her partner is so sensitive to stimuli, like touch or light or noise, they need to keep lights in the house dim, volume on the TV low or off. Though community seems important to both of them, they don't have family or friends over for fear of germs (he has become severely immunocompromised) and because the energy having guests requires knocks him out. She manages the home while continuing to work her office job remotely and spends a lot of time, she says, carrying things up and down stairs for him.

When we spoke again a year later, after his marriage proposal, she still didn't feel like the home was hers. She believed she could be disassociating from the house because, in her opinion, they needed to move: a move would allow her to be closer to family for support, and their current multi-story house was not accommodating to his needs. But what about hers? I mentioned that each time we spoke, she frequently brought up his needs or issues before her own. She confessed that their entire living situation is not what she had dreamt for herself:

> I grew up in the country and I loved just having wide open spaces and places for animals to run and wildlife. And now I'm just like, I need to be somewhere that's close to a hospital, a pharmacy, a grocery store. And so it's funny how your dreams change as you get older and you really learn to value the convenience of having medical care close by.

ALEXANDRA PICKED UP AND MOVED IN

The reality of cohabitating also flew in the face of Alexandra's expectations. She joined the ranks of the almost one in four Millennials who have moved back into a parent's home to provide care.[12] Alex didn't see it coming; she had to pick up and go. Terminal illness moves on its own timeline:

> When I said I'm moving home for "however long this takes," I think there's always a suspension of belief when you first hear such a shocking diagnosis. You hear the best-case scenario which, for glioblastoma, they'll say, like, five to seven years. So I was like, "Okay, I'm gonna move back to the States and be close to my mom for her last five to seven years," and I had no concept that meant that it was actually going to be fourteen months. There was some quality time, but it was so short. . . . She just had such [a] severe, severe case.

At the time of her mom's diagnosis, Alex had been living in Thailand for seven years; she ran her own company and had established a life there.

It was a life she quickly uprooted to get to her mom. She packed up everything in a week:

I had a dog that I had to get into the US, and I had a vet who was willing to forge the paperwork. Thank God. And I had a boyfriend at the time, too, and our relationship really was put to the test by the caretaking experience. We're not together anymore.... I couldn't handle the pressure of taking care of my mom and being in a relationship from afar.

It was a huge life adjustment, to say the least: it's a major transition to leave the life she built, her friends, her relationship, and she didn't have time to process. Meanwhile, she was dealing with the biggest upheaval: her mom had terminal brain cancer.

Once Alexandra arrived at her mom's home in upstate New York, her entire lifestyle changed. She provided her mom's full-time care until her stepdad's workday ended and they could share responsibilities at night. Her mom's care was no small undertaking: she was paralyzed within months of the diagnosis, required bed and wheelchair transfers, help bathing. Alex is active and fit—she used to be a diving instructor—but the job strained her body. Even with the help of a hired aide, she said caregiving was the most physically demanding thing she's ever done. She didn't see friends often; her life was devoted to her mom. Similar to Michelle's, this living situation created a rift in identity but, also, led to some important personal revelations:

For me caretaking was really eye-opening. I had never really tried that traditional life at all, of getting up and emptying the dishwasher and doing the laundry and doing those domestic tasks. And I think I always suspected that wouldn't be very satisfying for me, but I really found it more draining than I expected. And this was for my mom, who... there's no one that I love more in the world. So I just thought, if I can't find fulfillment doing this for her, I can really see very clearly [that] this is not my path in life. So some of the big

questions I'd been asking myself, like "do I want to have kids?" caretaking
really answered that for me pretty definitively.

KACI'S FIRST HOUSE, FOR MOM

By the age of thirty, Kaci had already bought and renovated her first
home—the sole reason was her mom's care. A parent moving in with
their adult child happens more often than we think, and in caregiving it's
quite common: of Millennials already caring for a parent, over a third of
them are providing the care in their own home.[13]

Kaci's care situation didn't begin that way: she had just moved abroad
to pursue a job as an au pair and her dream of living in another country, but shortly after arriving, her seemingly healthy mom underwent
emergency bypass surgery in upstate New York. Kaci returned home
right away. Over the next year unfolded a series of strokes, subsequent
surgeries, months in an ICU, and her mother's temporary move to a rehabilitation facility. Kaci's mom, still relatively young, required long-term
care—a move that needed to happen quickly. Kaci told me that the social
worker didn't complete her mother's paperwork, so her mom was moved
into a nursing home without a choice in where she was going. Kaci didn't
get to take a tour and had no voice in selection of her mom's new home or
care. Here's the thing about moving from a hospital or rehab to a live-in
care facility: the administration is shuffling patients from one location to
another, it's business they want to happen fast; for the patient and their
family, it's a decision of where that person *lives*. When she arrived to visit
her at the facility, Kaci was horrified. Her mom was on the floor, lying on
a mattress. Witnessing the level of neglect her mom was left in, Kaci made
it her job to be there and carry out the tasks her mom needed but wasn't
receiving care for:

She would call me crying, like "Please come put me to bed." I would have to
go put her to bed and that's why I really wanted her home, because I was just
spending every day in the nursing home. I would leave work at four o'clock,

go straight to the nursing home. Stay at the nursing home until midnight. Get her to bed, come back, and then that was my entire life.

It took the next year and a half, but Kaci was able to move her mother out. "It was my mission to buy a home, rehab the home, and get her out of there."

Buying a home, she said, was not something she would have otherwise done if not for the need to care for her mom herself. She had studied English as a Second Language (ESL) with the intention of living overseas. A home in Rochester, New York (where her mom lived), was never something she wanted. But now, on a teacher's income, she needed to make that happen. She had a very good credit score, her boyfriend at the time had money for the down payment—together they were viable homebuyers and were able to pull it off. It's a dream, buying a home, but Kaci said the reality of it annoyed her boyfriend, as did the money and construction required for renovations to accommodate her mother.

Though it afforded a lot of benefits, moving her mom in with her was not the end of complications—hardly. In New York state, you can't apply for medical grants (which can help pay for disability updates to a house) unless the care recipient has always lived at home; the move from the nursing facility made them ineligible. Five years after buying the house, she and her boyfriend broke up. She had to pay him back for the down payment, which, she said, "was really rough." Sharing a home is not an easy undertaking, particularly in a young adult's formative years. She was honest about how living with her mom influenced her dating life, her job prospects, and her mental health. Although she has the benefit of hired aides, she also said it can be uncomfortable to have strangers regularly in her home.

After we spoke, Kaci emailed me. Though she had spoken from her heart, there were some things that she wanted to clarify:

Sometimes when I talk about caregiving it takes me a minute to process everything I've been through, because my journey has been long. But at the end of the day, my mom is my best friend and I would be heartbroken to

*lose her. The months [she was] in the ICU were so painful for me because for
the first time in my life, I couldn't talk to my mom. Caregiving in my own
home has allowed me to actually be home.... The nursing home was worse
(because, yeah, terrible care) but also I was spending every evening and
weekend outside of work there. Having her home, while stressful at times,
has been an absolute blessing. Just to be able to sit on my couch with my dog
while my mom sits in her chair and we can watch TV.*

DEBBIE MOVED CLOSER AND MOM MOVED TO A FACILITY

About one in six Millennial caregivers cares for someone with dementia
and, of those caregivers, 84 percent do not live in the same household as
the person requiring care.[14] In her life before being a primary caregiver,
Debbie lived about a three-and-a-half-hour drive from her mom in Buffalo, New York, and was "doing her own thing." She says her mom was
pretty independent until a bad fall and its aftermath led to her mother's
dementia diagnosis.

Debbie's father passed away when she was very young, and her mother
never remarried: "It's her and I for a long, long time." That fall changed
things. Someone needed to step in and take a bigger role in ensuring her
mom's well-being, and Debbie knew that responsibility fell to her. She
"dropped everything" and took extended leave from her job to be with
her mom.

Debbie stayed with her mom for about six weeks and realized then the
trips home would need to be more frequent. Before dementia, she said,
she would go back home once every few months and for holidays. Now
she needed to be there a minimum of once a month to check in. Her mom
didn't want to leave her home—she had lived there for thirty years—and
didn't have any aides. Extended family and a few friends helped with
shopping and appointments:

*It was more of a group effort over those couple of years. I was still, I guess,
kind of the primary decision-maker, but doing that from afar, it was very*

helpful to have a couple of people in her life who were able to help with the
more practical day-to-day stuff that I just physically wasn't there for.

But Debbie knew traveling back and forth to Buffalo was not sustainable; after a couple of years, she moved there and moved her mom into independent living in the Buffalo area. About a year and a half later, she moved her mom into assisted living.

Assisted living facilities are not nursing homes, but still require an emotional adjustment. Because there is staff involvement in your family member's personal well-being and space, it forces you to face the fact that your loved one is no longer independent in the ways they used to be. I asked Debbie what that process was like for her.

It felt relieving. Because I just knew that she was in a building with other
people. And I realized there will be an adjustment period, getting used to the
routines and the staff and other residents, but I largely felt relieved about it.

Debbie's relief, as often does, also came with some guilt for the choice she'd made, despite knowing it was for the best:

My husband and I are somewhat recently married.... For me, kind of know-
ing the nature of my relationship with my mom and the distressing points
that we could get into at times, I felt like to preserve, protect my marriage
and have that part of my life not get wrapped up in the chaos, that my mom
living with us wasn't going to be, probably, the best option. I think there's
small bits of guilt about that sometimes. I certainly have watched other care-
givers, you know, move their parents in and I know it's... it's hard. I think
it's hard no matter what decision you make.

I've observed that, especially with caregiving, there's an instinct to compare your decisions to other people in similar roles or situations. Our care decisions are validated so infrequently, sometimes you look at someone who chose differently and think, "Wait, should I have done that?"

You question things, even the choices that are right for your family. A caregiver might judge themselves if their loved one moves into a facility; people not involved in the decision may even judge you as uncaring, unloving, undevoted. But I also knew that, in my family's case, there was no way I could have given my dad the level of care and attention he needed and still maintain our relationship in a healthy way. Still maintain my life, or his autonomy and independence from me, in a healthy way.

LONG-DISTANCE CAREGIVING

Long-distance caregivers know that it can still be a full-time job, but I also notice they sometimes undermine how much they do when comparing themselves to others. Because they didn't up and move, they may gloss over how much caregiving and illness impact their life when in conversation with other caregivers.

I'm still guilty of this at times. I was speaking with Jesus, who for years lived with both parents to support them financially and help care for his mom, who had diabetes, complications from a brain tumor, and then Parkinson's. When we spoke, his career had picked up and he was able to afford round-the-clock care for his mom and a place of his own. He lived less than a ten-minute drive away so he could check on them often. In the course of our conversation, I said, "I was a caregiver, but long distance." He picked up on the *but* and corrected me:

> It's caregiving, no matter if you're long distance or not. To your point, you said, "I was a caregiver, but long distance." It's like, as caregivers, we're so in our heads that we have to say that, but you know: yes, you were a caregiver. Are a caregiver.

The truth is, long-distance caregivers experience a lot of stress, they just experience it differently. When there was a hospital stay, I would also drop everything and go, but instead of getting in a car I was on a plane. It was expensive. If it wasn't an emergency, I had to ration out visits. Each time there was extended time off from the office, I was in New York. I wanted to be there, see my mom and friends too, but primarily be there *with him*. I wanted time with my dad and the relief of eyes on him to observe any small health or behavioral changes that needed addressing quickly and that maybe only a daughter could pick up on. When I was in California, I attempted to perceive changes over the phone; any difference in the way he sounded and I would pepper him with questions. Was his swallowing okay this week or worse? Can he handle thinner liquids again or does he choke? Then I'd ask my mom what she noticed: What was he like in person? Was there something we needed to do? If we didn't get ahead of a potential downturn, he might never recover. Often she would tell me, "If you could see him in person, you'd see it sounds worse than it is"; he was doing fine. *If I could see him in person.* The stress of not seeing him with my own eyes let my imagination do the diagnosing, which was rarely good.

Yet, many long-distance caregivers make it work. Years ago, before Alexa Show and Facebook tablets let you "drop in," my friend Brian told me about a system he devised to use Google's Remote Desktop to "appear" on his mom's computer screen. Brian was living in Mexico City, but his mom, who had advanced dementia and lived with Brian's blind father in New York, needed meal and medication reminders. (His brother and sister-in-law, and later hired aides, were also present and regularly on hand.) Using the remote desktop, his mother didn't even need to touch her computer for Brian to chat with her; it also allowed them to play games online and share photos. Since then, many technological advancements (including those directly aimed at elder tech and caregiving) have made long-distance caregiving logistically easier and safer.

Research on long-distance caregivers found they typically provide social and emotional support, advance care planning, financial assistance, and care coordination.[15] They often share responsibility with someone nearby who handles personal care. My advice to other long-distance caregivers rests on this cornerstone: have eyes and ears on the ground who can communicate with you, someone you trust who can accompany your loved one to doctor appointments and accurately relay information, someone (maybe the same person) who will visit your family member—to monitor the condition of their health and where they are living but also simply to share time with the person.

LONG-TERM CARE FACILITIES

In the course of your lifetime you'll come across at least one person who flippantly says, "I'd never put my [fill in name of loved one here] in a nursing home." To someone who has done it, or even considered it, it's insulting. Hurtful. The idea, the stigma, is that the decision to put someone out to pasture is made as casually as their comment; they don't know the considerations you weighed, the quality of care it's possible to receive, how that care can be better than you could have provided at home. They don't know that their words can reopen the wound made by the difficult decision in the first place, the pain of intimately witnessing the health condition that necessitated it, and that they can stoke guilt or defensiveness, even momentarily. I'm far from the only person who has felt this way.

One Caregiver Collective member said she got to a point when her mom's needs hit an intensity she could no longer handle safely on her own. She was physically unable to provide the care her mom needed and knew her mother needed to move to a nursing home, but she struggled with the widespread belief that nursing homes are "trash cans" for unloved seniors. The repeated refrain, that they are for people whose families don't love them, held her back. She felt guilty, even knowing it was the best decision for her mother's well-being.

Even with the COVID downturn, the United States has the largest number of nursing home residents in the world.[16] Care facilities are, as we live today, a fact of life and can be necessary. But the terrible stigma, and the pervasive guilt, persists. Another caregiver, who couldn't manage caring alone for her mom with brain cancer, said she "kicks herself" for not having the financial resources or a huge house that can accommodate her mom's medical needs. And to top that off: when you pay out of pocket, nursing homes are freaking expensive. Good care, bad care, any live-in care will wipe out savings.

Placing your parent in a nursing home is not indicative of how much you love them. I'm going to repeat that: *Placing your parent in a nursing home is not indicative of how much you love them.* Sometimes you cannot manage by yourself. Besides, some places can provide great care and sentiment. They become our de facto second homes. But they are not a replacement for family; you still must stay vigilant and watch everything like a hawk. At the end of the day, this is their business. They will make business choices you would not have chosen for your family, and it is up to you to prevent it. Bottom line. And some nursing homes are absolutely terrible. Kaci wasn't able to tour the nursing home before her mom was moved in and knew it was an important omission.

Kaci not only had that terrible experience with her mom's nursing home but also, when she tried to advocate for her mom, said they didn't take her seriously:

Of course I was the obnoxious one. And at times people treated me really crappy because of my age, and I would just [utilize] smoke and mirrors: I would bring a computer to every meeting and take notes on it so I looked important. But that nursing home, the things that I had to do....

If your person needs a care home, you need to tour it. Research ratings and reviews online. Once your family moves in, visit often. You need to inquire about everything and (politely, firmly) be the squeaky wheel so staff know not to mess with you. When they have parties, which my dad's home did often, go (not as an intimidation tactic but just for fun). Bring personal effects, decorate as you can. Let the staff know when you'll be calling or FaceTiming because for your loved one to even have their phone within reach or know to answer it when it rings can be a thing in itself.

With my dad's care, we also learned the importance of an *ombudsman* (I had no idea what this was either): ombudsmen are advocates in place at the nursing home to protect the residents' rights, advocate on residents' behalf, stop and prevent abuse, and hold staff accountable. They are there for you. Use them.

The takeaway from this chapter is this: a family's living situation, particularly when care is involved, should not be met with outside judgment. Instead, we should be focused on how to support the variety of living-with-care scenarios and work to ensure that every family has the access and ability to make the decision best for them.

CHAPTER 5

WHY ISN'T MY SIBLING HELPING? AND OTHER FAMILY DYNAMICS

The biggest challenge [with] the Parkinson's...has been actually with the other people in the family.... It's when there's betrayals. And people won't step up. And people make excuses for literal years to not help.

—Brandon, 40

AN ASPIRING WRITER FROM MICHIGAN, BRANDON WAS IN HIS EARLY thirties and attending grad school in New York when his mother's condition became worrisome. He describes his younger self as driven, determined, ambitious. Even states away, he observed changes in his mom's behavior and condition: she'd lost a significant amount of weight, didn't look healthy, and had become afraid to drive. He questioned what was going on. She was sleeping more, could she have depression? "From afar, I was piecing together what I could, and I knew things were different." He says her condition at that time was "spiraling."

Brandon is now forty, the middle of three brothers. His older brother worked for their mom at the time and saw her every day; Brandon begged this brother to get more involved in keeping an eye on their mother but was met with a combination of denial and resentment. Brandon also admits to his own denial at the beginning ("We felt too young for all this....I was in my early thirties. Mom was in her late fifties"), but he couldn't ignore her obvious decline. Doctors went through rounds of varying diagnoses and prescriptions until they finally landed on Parkinson's. It became clear someone needed to step in and be there, to get his mom situated with a new normal of living with disease. He thought once the doctor appointments were taken care of and a medicine regimen established, she could continue living on her own. It would only take a couple of months.

His older brother wouldn't do it. He was in the middle of a divorce at the time and dealing with alcoholism; he blatantly refused to help. Brandon had a better relationship with his younger brother, who was in his late twenties and also lived in New York. Before, they'd been close. "We'd always been able to count on each other, kind of being there for certain emotional needs and all that stuff. And I think that the caregiving changed that." His brother traveled a lot for work; his schedule wasn't as flexible as Brandon's. They discussed sharing future care coordination, maybe even moving their mom closer to New York, but for now Brandon seemed like the natural choice to go to Michigan. Brandon also said his connection with his mom, her emotional support for him over the years, influenced his decision to be there for her.

Brandon didn't expect that when he arrived the situation would continue to spiral. "It was about a year of just endless tests and experimental treatments and exploratory surgery and all these things to try to figure out what was this debilitating pain that had started with her." It became evident that his move back in with his mother would become permanent. "It was just clear, 'Yeah, the old life was over'... somewhere along those lines I just realized, 'Okay, you're not going back to New York.'"

He became the boots on the ground, coordinating doctor appointments and medications, attending support groups, researching the disease and anything that could help, learning what to expect. Brandon shared this information with his younger brother to get him on the same page but felt the information and his observations of their mom, his opinions, weren't heard. It led to a lot of resentment toward his younger brother:

I had done all the work, I had made the sacrifices. I had gone to Michigan for years where we grew up and where I left. I did hundreds of hours of doctor's appointments and support groups and taking her to physical therapy and specialized physical therapy. And I gained all this knowledge and then he wouldn't listen to me when we got here. And I'd be asking him, like, can you help with recipes? And then he's telling me about how he doesn't have time, or he has a job, and these condescending things. And I understand that it's denial and all these things, but it was this, "Okay, so I have completely rerouted my entire life and I'm asking you the easiest things and you're telling me that you don't have time for it."...Everything turned into this negotiation.

Brandon doesn't think the resentment is one-way. He admits that energy and attention he would have spent on interest in his brother's life was instead diverted to their mom's care, and he believes his brother harbors resentment at their changed relationship. Brandon was also, let's face it, pissed that his brother's personal life continued: "I did have resentments for his normal life going on. And I know those early years of caregiving, I'm sure I stopped asking about 'how are personal projects going?' and 'how is work going?' Because I didn't want to hear about it. I wish I had a normal job. I wish I had more time for my [own interests].... I didn't want to hear about his normal job, but I can see how that would be perceived as taking less interest." Particularly because he believes his younger brother was in denial about their mom's condition, Brandon understands how his emotional absence could've been misunderstood and misinterpreted.

Misunderstanding was at the root of a lot of what Brandon shared about his relationship with his younger brother. "I can think of a number of our fights that were motivated by me being angry. He didn't understand that...I have these goals. And I wanted him to come for a couple weeks so I could have a couple of weeks to work on my stuff.... I guess I just feel overlooked in that way."

To make matters worse, Brandon worried that his older brother had dipped into their mother's savings, and he had concerns over mismanagement of her company's funds, suspecting it had depleted money for her retirement and care. The financial situation, he says, put extra pressure on him and his younger brother and also affected their relationship. The situation underscored for him that if you have a sibling you couldn't trust before caregiving, such as his older brother, don't start trusting them now. The care situation only exacerbates who people have always been, the roles they've already assumed.

Brandon has been able to figure out how to care for his mom, but he hasn't been able to fill her shoes. He says the dynamic between the brothers also suffered in the absence of their mom's usual interventions to keep the family together. Still, Brandon has hope for his relationship with his younger brother, who is now trying to wrap his head around what care for their mom looks like. When I asked Brandon if he wishes he had handled things differently with his younger brother, he said, "Of course. I do wish I could have figured out how to be more gentle and to communicate more and explain more, even if I shouldn't have had to.... [Caregiving] does bring out those [sibling] dynamics, although at the same time, that was the thing I resented, too, because I wish I had a big brother who...would explain to me what I needed to do.... To me, that has been the defining thing of this, is losing the shape of our whole family."

CAN'T WE ALL BE ON THE SAME PAGE?

It is often that one sibling takes on more, if not most, of the caregiving burden of an elderly parent. A study by the Alzheimer's Association found 61 percent of siblings felt they didn't get the support they needed from their brothers and sisters and it strained their relationships.[1] As an only child who dreamt of having siblings to share care with, this blew my mind. Lea was the first caregiver who punctured my fantasy. One of seven kids, she's the only one to take on daily responsibility for her parents' care, even moving across states and uprooting her husband and young child to do so. She explained it as a combination of denial and unwillingness on her siblings' parts (sound familiar?).

After Kaci's mom had a stroke, she went to live with Kaci's older brother. It lasted about a month: "He was just like, 'I can't.'" Her mom eventually moved into the house Kaci purchased to prevent her from going back into a nursing home; her brother visits on Sundays to give Kaci a reprieve. "If I ask him to stay over or something once in a while, he'll do it. But it's hard. Mom didn't even want him taking her to the bathroom." The tasks he does take on require Kaci to write out a plan for him because she's the only one who knows what to do for their mom hour by hour.

Members in my group often voice the resentment that grows while they watch their siblings build the lives they want without consideration for the caregiver, and how families can be ripped apart by feelings of abandonment, selfishness, and misunderstanding. Some caregivers I interviewed said their sibling relationships have become so tumultuous as a result of caregiving that they wouldn't talk about it on the record, even knowing names would be changed. There are mental health implications to this: during the pandemic, the CDC found that caregivers who had experienced caregiving-related family disagreements or who resented their caregiving responsibilities were three times more likely to report adverse mental health symptoms than other caregivers.[2]

When multiple siblings are involved with caregiving, there can still be issues. Members of the Collective have posted about sibling rivalry when it comes to proxy designation ("she's Dad's favorite, let her handle it"). A good friend, one of three sisters, recently told me how difficult it's been for the siblings to agree on care for their mom, who has Alzheimer's. Although my friend is the only one geographically present with their mother, seeing the situation with her own eyes, her sisters have strong opinions. They try to make unanimous decisions, but she feels her sisters don't have a realistic grasp of the situation, despite their wholehearted concern. They're in different places in their lives, and they are coming at the problem from different perspectives. There isn't animosity, but there is frustration.

When it comes to siblings not offering the same level of involvement you might, or who are just not on the same page, Christina Irving, social worker at Family Caregiver Alliance, says a family meeting facilitated by a third party (like a therapist or social worker) can be helpful. "Sometimes having that neutral third-party person, or somebody who's viewed as a professional [and] knows what they're doing, that [person] can be heard in a way that the actual caregiver may not be heard."

THERE *ARE* SIBLINGS WHO TACKLE CAREGIVING TOGETHER, AS "TEAM-mates." That's how Laura phrased it when we sat in her living room while her infant son was at day care. Laura is one of my oldest friends; she experienced caregiving for her dad after mine had already passed. She and her older brother, Mike, cared for their dad through years of dementia and, finally, unexpectedly, late-stage cancer and the chemo that accompanied it. Having known both Laura and Mike since adolescence, I didn't see that caregiving had torn them apart. Now more than a year after their dad's death, I wondered how she looked back on the experience with her brother. "We had always had a close relationship, but this made us stronger people individually and then, I think, gave us more intense respect for each other. It made us closer in certain ways."

From my conversations with Laura, it seemed that what made the difference was a like-minded approach on decision-making and a willingness to tag team. They divvied up responsibilities, managing plans together but executing separately. When one person needed a reprieve, the other would step up. She told me about a time during the COVID Omicron surge, when their dad was in the hospital at his sickest from chemo: "There was a one-person [visitor] cap per day...it was a saving grace that Mike and I were sharing the care because we switched off each day. And I was taking care of, at the time, an almost one-year-old, so I just couldn't go every day....I counted on him going, knowing that when I went, he would go the next day. That tag team was very crucial."

Laura and Mike weren't just a tag team, they were each other's confidants. She was a new mom, he was going through a divorce. They grappled with the declining health of their dad, who they were both close to, as well as decisions about which medical interventions to attempt. Both were emotionally and physically, well, spent. "I would get so miserable after having a frustrating conversation with Dad and I would call Mike and he'd be the only one who would understand the minutiae of it all. And there's nothing like that. Nothing compares, in a way, to somebody you don't have to update all the time, you don't have to catch up." At the end of a long day, they could laugh together about what she called that day's medical "absurdities" and lean quietly on each other. They knew each other's tells, they intentionally tried not to stress the other one out. *This* is the sibling fantasy I was talking about.

Though they were in it together, the heft of the situation didn't always fall equally. The different relationships they each had with their father played a role, and Laura believes gender played a part. Early in their dad's illness, Laura admits it was Mike who shouldered the most responsibility: he was the first to notice changes in their dad's behavior and to bring it up to the doctors he and their dad shared. Despite the siblings' synchronization on decision-making (Laura says she and her brother joke they are "mind-melded"), they had different outlooks. She felt like her brother was clinging to the "old dad" to try to keep the father they knew for as long as possible, while she was practicing the long journey of letting go and just trying to enjoy time with him. As the dementia progressed, Mike was given power of attorney (POA). At the time, Laura said their dad wanted Mike's help with particular things, despite her willingness to be involved. She believes some of it was logistical, because Mike had POA and, at first, was the lead coordinating with doctors, but also because their dad felt more comfortable discussing men's health with his son. She thinks her dad wanted to preserve his sense of dignity, particularly in front of women, even his daughter. Being the younger girl of the family, even as adults, still played a part. For a time, Laura believed their dad didn't trust her with his care the same way he trusted her brother and that he took Mike more seriously as the older sibling. "He treated me like a daughter, [in] an old-fashioned 'I was still a baby' kind of way."

Eventually, the responsibility on Mike was too significant and gradually Laura took on more of an equal role. "Stuff has been on Mike's plate that has been so overwhelming that he has suffered, definitely…it was too much to handle. And I started over a course of five to seven years learning all the doctors. I started going because I remember Mike saying, 'If you could go to some of these appointments, that'd be helpful.' And I did, I started learning all that." Her dad was receptive. "I feel like in the end, he did trust us both…when we would go to the hospital, he would say [to staff] things like, 'Make sure you tell her, make sure you tell everything to her.'"

OLD FAMILY PATTERNS REAR AGAIN

Like Laura, I also felt there were times my dad still saw me as a little girl. Truthfully, I cherished the feeling. It worked to undo some of the role reversal I had taken on in watching out for him. It was a comfortable role for me and, I think, stoked warm childhood feelings of safety and paternal protection.

Michelle found herself playing out a different type of outdated familial pattern, a dynamic of behavior passed down to her—one that she wasn't altogether comfortable with. Parental expectations can feel imposing, even when you're in your thirties—and especially when you're living at home as Michelle was and where her parents' authority still felt supreme. Michelle felt the model set in her family was to give selflessly to her mom, even at personal expense; it was a pattern her dad adopted for himself, an expectation he transposed onto Michelle. However, she felt like she was the only one making large personal sacrifices. She navigated sharing care responsibilities with her dad, who she refers to as her "care partner," while trying to delegate to her mom tasks Michelle thought she was able to handle; but Michelle felt she was the one wrestling the most to make accommodations. It was the impossible balance of her mom's needs with Michelle's work hours and deadlines that finally broke the camel's back. Morning doctor appointments for her mom meant Michelle often arrived late to the office, then worked late hours to compensate. She was exhausted. "It was almost like I was a little bit in denial of what that situation [her mom's escalating illness] meant and what I would have to change. It was just horrible for all of us. And there was no sense of how do we try to, as a family, get out of this a little bit? And ultimately, it was me adjusting my schedule that made it tenable." Michelle took family medical leave. In retrospect, she wished her parents could see where they could've given a bit, too, to help her cope.

Michelle's family is also "pretty private," which meant they did not share details about her mom's illness with extended family. This placed more weight on Michelle by eliminating a potential support system she could have leaned on, "which made it also really difficult to ask for help when others weren't fully aware of the whole health situation and how bad it had gotten." So many of my talks with Michelle came down to her wanting, needing, help and feeling unanswered in that hope. And again, this was Michelle following the preexisting dynamic set by her parents. Even as an adult kid, especially one living in our parents' home, we can feel helpless to change the dynamic we grew up with. The parents are still The Parents.

Setting boundaries when it comes to caregiving, especially when you're emulating a familial behavioral pattern, is difficult.

"That's the challenge of caregiving...it often exacerbates some of the existing family dynamics and what that relationship is," Christina Irving says. "If you had a really either close relationship or maybe a parent that was a little bit more strict and set the roles and guidelines, it's that much harder to set your own boundaries and to have yourself as an adult with your own identity and your own needs in that relationship." It can be made even more difficult, she says, when the care recipient has high expectations for you providing their care; your boundaries may require changing a situation that has been working out well for them, at your expense. So *how* can we approach setting boundaries?

Start by remembering your own value and worth. Irving says it's important to help caregivers "realize your own needs are valuable and important to you as a person outside of your role as a caregiver. Just as a person, you have value and importance and worth....And yes, there are moments where you're going to have to prioritize what they need, but it should not be every moment."

When it comes to these kinds of boundary-setting conversations, "earlier is better," Irving says, though she realizes that if care comes on suddenly, it may take a little while to see what the reality looks like. She recommends, when approaching your care recipient with your needs, to treat them as "a partner in problem-solving this." You can frame your concerns by saying, "I am here for you, I want to support you and help make sure that you are cared for and your health is as good as it can be. There are also things that I need to be able to do for myself, and so sometimes I'm not going to be able to be here as much as you would like me to, and we may need to look at other options and who else can be involved." She recommends empathy and understanding for the other person's situation, while being assertive in standing up for yourself. The other person may not want to hear your concerns or to change their behavior; the process requires consistency on your part to uphold your needs. "A lot of that comes down to individual work that the caregiver ends up having to do and getting support around that, either from peers [or] a support group, from friends, from a counselor. Because it's a hard thing to do."

FAMILY WHO THINK THEY KNOW BEST

Then there's the extended family who just don't get it. Earlier I mentioned Mia, the full-time caregiver for her best friend, a vet who suffers from multiple traumatic injuries and PTSD. They planned a trip to visit his immediate family, something she was looking forward to; finally, she'd have other people around who could help her and she could relax a bit. Instead, she found that his family misses the "old" him and downplays his injuries and the intensity of care required; she feels their neglect endangers his safety and health. They expect his condition is temporary and he will "get better," an outcome Mia and her best friend both know isn't in the cards.

Denial isn't the only reason some family members don't comprehend the severity of illness and the lengths to which the caregiver is going to manage health. Every time I speak with Casey, who cares for her now-husband, it's clear how close she is with her family. She considers her mom her best friend and, since her parents moved abroad, has replaced visits with regular phone calls. In-person connection to the rest of her family, including sisters and extended family who live nearby, had been restricted since the pandemic when her husband's illness began. Family visits wear her husband out easily and have long-lasting effects on his fatigue. There aren't many precautions taken around him because she finds her family don't truly understand his "invisible illness." Casey thinks conveying the severity of his illness to them is particularly tough because, when he does see other people, he tries to come off as happy and healthy, "always trying to not drag the group down." On one Thanksgiving visit to her grandparents' home, she instructed her husband (then-boyfriend) not to pretend to be healthier than he is. Casey knew if her family saw him seemingly "normal" and happy, they would think nothing was wrong; they'd have a better grasp of his situation if they could see his actual condition for themselves.

Connecting with more extended family seems to be something Casey doesn't put much faith in, thinking it may lead to more headache than help:

> We actually haven't told that many of our more extended friends or family…we're just kind of afraid to talk publicly about it because everyone's gonna have certain stigmas that are attached to that, right? Immediately they're gonna be like, "Well, have you tried yoga? Have you tried diets? Have you tried essential oils? Have you tried not being sick?"…A lot of people just don't know how to respond.…They haven't been caretakers themselves. I don't think they understand the situation well.

Christina Irving suggests acknowledging that these uncomfortable conversations are going to happen, and it doesn't necessarily mean anything about the quality of care you're providing:

> When you get those comments…take that deep breath for a second. I think some of it is fighting against being defensive. I think caregivers often want to

justify, "No, I'm doing it right." And sometimes that comes from those worries
that a lot of caregivers have: "Am I doing it right?" You're there, so that right
there is more than those other family members are doing because you are
actually the one who is there and doing it.... Remembering that [is import-
ant], being able to acknowledge that for yourself. Sometimes getting that
acknowledgment, validation from others is really helpful in shoring up your
ability to not feel railroaded by those other family members.

BUILDING NEW FAMILY DYNAMICS—AND REDISCOVERING CHERISHED OLD ONES

In Alexandra's family, she was the sibling who uprooted to move back in
and care all day for her mom, who had brain cancer. It was clear that caring for her mother had taxed Alexandra heavily, but in our conversation
I was struck by the cast of care characters she referenced: her stepdad,
who also lived in the house, was involved with her mom's care when he
wasn't at work; her sister, who lived out of state, visited often on weekends
or when she had a break from her job; even her dad (her mom's longtime
ex-husband) flew out twice to stay in the house with her stepdad so Alex
could attend a work event or a friend's wedding. But beyond the immediate family, there were her mom's friends, who provided additional support. "We had a huge, incredible community, which was really helpful.
My mom had friends coming from every direction that really wanted to
help us and so that felt amazing and supportive.... My mom did have one
best friend... and I did call her in some emergencies when I was home
alone and I needed someone on speed dial who could show up and could
help. And I can't imagine doing it without that."

When Alexandra mentioned her dad arriving to help, I recognized a
theme: When Laura and her brother needed to clean out their dad's apartment, their mom (his ex-wife) showed up to help. Brandon's parents had
been divorced since he was in the sixth grade, but with his mom's diagnosis, "even my dad... stepped up in this situation to help out and he's been

a support from afar. He lives in northern Michigan, but people do rise up and come together, and you learn strengths and things that you didn't have." I lived this in my own family. When I was in Los Angeles, my mom escorted my dad to doctor appointments. She visited him in the nursing home, always with a cupcake or my dad's favorite Dunkin' donut, and she'd sit with him for meals and activities; he always had family around. One afternoon I took my dad to the movies. I'd preplanned everything for what was, once, a spontaneous activity: the accessible ride, a theater that had accommodations for wheelchairs, my purse was packed with bendy straws and a can of the thickened protein shakes he could swallow. After the movie, I parked my dad's wheelchair in the lobby while I ran into the restroom. When I returned minutes later, I spotted him and my spidey sense immediately went up: a woman, bent beside his chair, was chatting my dad up. She was a grifter, I knew it, who'd spotted a vulnerable older man and was greasing him for bank account details. He loved women, he would fall for it; I needed to plan our extraction. As I got closer, I realized: it was *my mom*. She had been in the area, knew what time the movie let out, and had come to meet us.

My mom joined me for a lot of visits, and my dad began coming over to spend holidays with us. When the three of us once stopped at a bakery on Bleecker Street, my dad and I sat outside while my mom went in and I told him how pissed I was at her that day for this or for that. My dad, in his wisdom and knowledge of women, had one message for me: "Leave me out of it." This moment between us felt *normal*. It was a family dynamic I'd never expected to rediscover with my divorced parents. It felt as though we'd somehow been reshaped back to how we began, all present as a unit. Most of all, it taught me a lot about marriage and family before being married myself. Despite their past, once they shared a daughter, that was it: family for life. My mom showed up for my dad, and me, when it wasn't easy but when it really mattered.

Am I suggesting all divorced parents resolve past pain when caregiving shows up? No. But be open to the unexpected. The presence of illness or aging could provide an opportunity to resolve past pains. New dynamics will emerge that you don't expect—don't discount that the relationship you have with family will be one of them, and that it could be for the good.

When it comes to extended family, my takeaways from the Collective are that you may be pleasantly surprised by their involvement; try to lean into the possibility that family may have helpful suggestions, or emotional support, at the ready. They may be willing to learn more about the disease or step in with practical help, like sending over a cooked meal or helping with laundry. Casey, who experiences family challenges, did tell me that her husband's aunt had been a caregiver and shared a tip on adaptive cutlery. "It's not a huge game changer, but it's a little bit of help that he didn't have before and that's something I never would have thought of."

CHAPTER 6

ROMANTIC RELATIONSHIPS ARE HARD AND WILL I GET TO HAVE KIDS?

MAYBE IT'S NO SURPRISE THAT THE MOST LIVE PARTICIPATION IN A Caregiver Collective webinar was on romantic relationships. If building a partnership or a family isn't a priority, it's at least a point of reflection, possible decision, or, worst, unsolicited conversation. When you're the current age of Millennials and without a partner or children, it can feel super shitty when someone asks when you're going to get married or start a family. The implication is you're behind or have given up entirely. For Millennials at the receiving end of "when are you getting married, having kids, living up to my expectations" *and also caregiving*, the questions are extra loaded. We're in the years considered by many to be prime to partner up and procreate and *we feel it*; but we're also busy and don't know how to initiate a relationship while keeping the wheels from falling off the caregiving. When we think of caregiving within the family context, naturally thoughts zero in on the family member in need of care— but what about the families we are still in the process of building?

Millennial caregivers often don't experience the same dating opportunities as other young adults, and they already feel socially disadvantaged and removed from their peers. In one online support chat, a member voiced how they dreaded the upcoming holidays because it meant seeing extended family. At the time, he was in his late thirties, unmarried, and had been caring for his mom for years. He knew family members would ask about his dating life, expressing their expectations for him to start a family. The thought of it enraged him. How could they think he had time or energy to meet someone when they never offered help or support to care for his mom? A fellow group member fielded this line of questioning on marriage from *her insurance agent*. There are also those who assume you've already put yourself out to pasture. Another caregiver in her thirties shared that a family friend told her, "Thank goodness you are never getting married so you can always take care of your mom." The comments on that post lit up in her defense.

Caregiving directly informs the social opportunities we have to find partners, the decisions we make when building families in light of caregiving (from the partners we choose to the number of kids we decide to have), or if we do it at all. We weigh the same considerations as our peers but also how the person we care for and those responsibilities fit into the equation. Or better said: how our own partners and families can fit around caregiving.

So, believe that when sex and relationship therapist Dr. Lisa Paz offered to speak directly to us in a webinar about how to date and maintain romantic relationships as a caregiver our age, members tuned in. People have questions; raising these questions exposes a myriad of valid fears: that we're not going to have the opportunity to pursue the dreams and expectations we had for ourselves, that we can't financially or emotionally sustain supporting our own family, that we'll be alone, that no one will care for us. When caregiving feels like it dictates dating or family planning in a way that dashes our deepest hopes, it can add another layer of ambiguous loss for the life you "thought" you'd have.

SOME STATISTICAL TRUTH: WHEN IT COMES TO MARRIAGE, UNMARRIED caregiving Millennials aren't far behind their peers. Millennials marry and have children later than previous generations did.[1] Our generation is having kids, just not necessarily when we were told to. Many women today are becoming first-time mothers in their forties.[2] In 2018, US women were waiting longer but also were more likely to have children than a decade ago.[3]

A Pew Research Center article states that Millennials "have been slower than previous generations" to start families, that we "trail behind previous generations at the same age." Even this language implies a standard not being met. In some ways, that's true: we came upon family-building age at a time of economic insecurity and even devastation. Between multiple economic downturns and student loan debt, it may take longer to position ourselves in a financially secure place to start a family; we often consider whether we can even afford to have kids. Our parents' generation didn't face the same societal obstacles. Our illusions of their standard long ago broken, our expectations are more malleable. Given current economic conditions, the trend of having children later seems likely to continue.[4]

But financial reasons are not the only factor in play when explaining why we're building families later. Emphasis on building a career may delay when we have kids. Fertility options are marketed to us through social media the moment we hit our mid-twenties, informing us that waiting can be a viable (although expensive) option. And guess what, some people just choose not to have kids.

For a caregiver, having a partner may not be just about having children, or someone to spend your time with, an intimate connection. Look, those are big things. Songs and stories have been devoted to this for centuries. But it's also about having someone close to you who can help. Someone who can see and understand intimately what you're going through, maybe take some off your plate. In even more unromantic terms, caregiving is expensive. A single person taking that on alone while also self-financing their life is daunting. I told you it's not romantic, but it's a real thought some caregivers have.

This is not my stump speech in favor of traditional marriage, or even partnership. But I do wonder, for those who wanted to partner early in life but didn't as a result of being a caregiver, if there will be larger repercussions for our generation.

DOES CAREGIVING IMPACT OUR ROMANTIC RELATIONSHIPS? EASY: YES. But how *exactly*? And, when it's negative, what can we do about it? Let's break this down into phases of romantic relationships and family building.

WHEN YOU'RE DATING (IF YOU'RE DATING)

I grieve a lot of my adolescence, my twenties and my early thirties. When most people are dating, looking for a partner or looking for someone to settle down with, looking to build a family, I was not doing that, frankly. I was surviving financially, mentally, emotionally with this experience. So only now…I've woken up to so much of the years…that part of my life that I've lost. But now I'm more open about what I want.

Ron is a polished guy in his early forties, an attorney in New York working in finance. In objective terms, Ron is a catch. But for the majority of his life, Ron's love life was affected by caring for his mom who, you'll remember, has psychiatric mental illness and dementia. He describes himself as being her primary financial, logistical, and emotional caregiver since he was sixteen or seventeen, and her live-in caregiver for a decade. Despite wanting a family of his own, he says the experience preyed upon his doubt that it could ever be a possibility.

A lot of people can relate to the acute angst that they may never have the partner or family they dreamt of for themselves. That feeling can be terrible enough, but for Ron it is echoed by his family…including his mom. The woman whose need for care dictated where Ron lived, went to college, and who he lived with also wanted to impress on him that she wanted him to be partnered.

"That's all she knew. She got married when she was twenty-something, she never knew life without a spouse and doesn't believe in life without a spouse. So every day I hear that. There's not a day that goes by that I [don't] hear something about, 'When are you going to settle down? Have you found someone yet? Don't live life alone.'" Although it comes from a place of love, her own wishes for her son to be loved and taken care of, it feels like another insurmountable ask. Making it feel worse: Ron agrees. "[She's] sharing really good morsels of wisdom, there's truth to it. Sharing life's burdens is helpful."

In his twenties and thirties, the subconscious belief that he would never be able to meet someone his age who could understand his life at home, or would want to, held Ron back from being honest about his desires for partnership. Now in his forties, Ron acknowledges those feelings and actually sees an advantage to dating at this age as a caregiver: "As I've aged through the caregiving process, it feels more possible that when you do meet someone, they can understand a little bit more of the situation. They've grown up a little bit more, they've reached a level of maturity in their own life, there's a little bit more connectedness between you and another person." He says it's given him hope. He's honest with himself and voices his wants openly. He sees it as a major step in living authentically.

Is Dating Even Possible When Someone Else Is My Priority?

This is a predominant question among single caregivers. I think the quick answer people tell themselves is "no" so that joining dating apps and putting themself out there isn't another thing on the to-do list to stress over. You may ask yourself what you can viably offer and whether someone else would see your situation as baggage. When a caregiver is ready, and truly wants it, questions take on the logistical aspects of finding the time and energy to date.

Ron openly admitting that he wants to settle down was a big first step, an emotional accomplishment. Now he finds that dating conflicts with where he is physically and emotionally as a caregiver. "I try to fit in a date when I can.... You're caught between this rock and this hard place of wanting a life for yourself that you always dreamed of...while at the same time you butt up against burnout and exhaustion from caregiving for the last twenty-some-odd years, that relationships become hard and difficult. They take energy and commitment and investment that you sort of gave already. To go and give that again is a choice, and I'm willing to make it, but it's difficult."

Adrienne was caregiving for her mom when she posted, "I consider dating just one more thing to juggle, but you know I did it last year when I was in a relationship and I WILL DO IT AGAIN. I also don't waste my time on people I'm interested in for the sake of dating just to date…ain't nobody got time for that!"

Talking to Kaci about her attitude toward dating was a 180; her situation is also completely different. Kaci had just entered into a new relationship when her mom had a stroke. "It kind of fast-tracked the relationship….We probably wouldn't have worked out, but because my mom got sick, it was all of a sudden like all hands on deck." Her former partner helped Kaci care for her mom until their relationship ended five years later. In contrast to Ron, when Kaci entered caregiving right away it existed simultaneously with a relationship; maybe not well, but it was possible. When the relationship ended, Kaci was open to dating again. "I was sitting at home and I started assessing my situation and I was like, 'Oh my gosh, I'm thirty-three years old and here I am sitting at home with my mom on a Friday night. This is gonna get bad, fast.' So I went on the dating apps like people do and he [her current boyfriend] was probably like my third or fourth date….I was using it [dating] as a way to just get out and meet people my age because I was just around my mom all the time."

After Kaci explained navigating relationships and dating with her full care and career schedules, my big question for her was: *How?*

She told me that she relied on aides so that she was able to leave the house to go on dates. "He jokes about it now, because he thought I was Cinderella because at like 10:50 p.m. I was like, I gotta get home. And he didn't know that I had an aide waiting for me. He didn't understand that at the time. Now he totally gets it." When she and her boyfriend spend time together now, it's planned for the days when aides are already scheduled to be with her mom. She believes he's gotten used to the routine of it.

Her system is far from flawless or without unplanned interruptions that require Kaci to jump in, but it's provided her some breathing room for a personal life. (I notice a lot of caregivers think they can't afford or have access to aide services. Kaci pays for aides through a New York state Medicaid program. It's an imperfect system we get into later in the book, but I want to raise here the possibility that aides may be covered by insurance.)

For advice, I again reached out to Dr. Lisa, who has experience working with family caregivers. She agreed that stepping into dating as a caregiver can be daunting: "Early courtship behavior is [saying], 'I am going to put out the shiniest best version of myself and really peacock out.' And if you can't access that shiniest best version of yourself, then it can feel really overwhelming." Although it may feel difficult, dating can be an act of connecting to other pieces of yourself, preserving those aspects of your identity.

Worrying about what you have available to bring to the table and those thoughts keeping you from getting into a relationship can be forms of self-sabotage, she says.

> Sometimes we project our insecurities, or what we see as our shortcomings, onto potential suitors. We're like, "I want to protect them from my stuff. I don't want to bring anyone into this." But in doing that, we're doing the work for them.... They need to decide. Maybe they have abundant capacity. Maybe you're delightful and special and sexy and fabulous enough that they have room to take it on. By [asking] this question of "shouldn't we ask ourselves what we are offering?" what I hear is, "shouldn't we let them know that we have limitations that are really going to interrupt this?" And no, I don't think that's your work. I think that's their work to assess if they want to take it on or not after you show up as your authentic self.

She advises single caregivers thinking about dating to ask what they are seeking for themselves outside of caregiving:

> People [should] be asking themselves, why aren't they dating? Do they want a partner? Because I think that there are people that are like, "I'm not

looking for this just because everyone at Thanksgiving is [asking] why hav-en't you found someone?" They need to be asking, do I want someone in the first place? But I think if the answer is yes, I would love to be dating or in love or I would love to be facilitating this part of my identity...it's a good enough reason to at least play with the idea in spite of the fact that it will require extra effort and you're exhausted and it's going to have to be making time and there might be [hesitation around] that up-front piece of when do you disclose that you are a primary caregiver and what that means.

When Do You Bring Up Caregiving with a Date?

I've noticed people take different tactics when deciding how soon to tell a date that they're a caregiver. Kaci told her boyfriend early on—the sec-ond date—that she was caring for her mom. They lived in different states at the time and she didn't really think the date would lead anywhere, so didn't feel much pressure. Members of the Collective have debated the dilemma of mentioning caregiving in a dating app profile; is it best to leave it out, or would including the information filter out potential dates who would be turned off by their situation? When Adrienne was trying to date while caring for her mom, she didn't lead with that information. Adrienne posted, "I go on dates here and there but just like big things in your life that you don't reveal right away (unless you're on *The Bachelor*), I don't bring it up immediately...especially if it's not someone I'm inter-ested in. That said, sometimes I get a bit nervous about how they react but also know the RIGHT guy will embrace it and understand."

Jessica was caring for both parents long distance, intimately involved in their care and visiting often. She met her boyfriend on Bumble, and they've been together for seven years. "Honestly, I kept the whole relation-ship under wraps for probably the first three to four months. I think it's one thing to tell someone my mom/dad/grandparent has XYZ diagnosis, but it's a whole other thing to live it and experience it." Once they got to know each other better, she learned her boyfriend's dad had been living with a rare blood cancer for over twenty years. "The right person would be willing and understanding to just go with the flow because you never know what will happen."

Dr. Lisa says there is no hard-and-fast rule of when to disclose you're a caregiver, that it's case by case and what feels right to you. She reminded me that, at the beginning, dating should be light and fun; the first date is a checkpoint to see whether you want to spend more time with this person, so there's no need to lay everything out up front. When it comes to what to include in your app profile, "I would love to see people lead with who they are apart from caregiver or in addition. Not because it's anything negative, but because it's not your entirety…there's so many different pieces to us and [to] over-lead with any one thing is a disservice to someone getting to know you."

Ask yourself what you want to lead with: your profession, where you grew up, your favorite kind of music or how you like to spend a Sunday. And if including caregiving as part of your profile feels like it best describes you, do it. Dr. Lisa says:

> *Neither is right or wrong. I think it's about people figuring out what feels like their authentic narrative, but I don't think [including caregiving in a profile] should be a caution sign…it's not fair. I think they're undercutting themselves. You're a caregiver among a million other things and the people that are going to like you are going to see the purity in it, the beauty in it, the pain in it, the responsibility in it, all that it is. But putting it into a dating profile because you're weeding people out? You're not weeding anyone out. You're protecting them from your insecurity about what this is or you're overidentified with [the role] or you're afraid [of rejection] or you haven't figured out how to say, "I'm a writer who lives in Berlin and grew up in New York and I love Chinese food and sushi on Sundays, and I'm a caregiver."*

Should I Date Another Caregiver?

It could make sense to date another caregiver, right? Someone on a similar path who can relate to a shared emotional experience that not everyone understands. Similar family priorities can be a draw, as is not having to explain why you may be canceling last minute. Another caregiver would get it. Dr. Feylyn Lewis, the caregiving researcher, has observed that young adult caregivers tend to romantically partner with people who "either needed care or were caregivers themselves." "That messiness of life is more accepted," she said. "You're not ashamed of it because somebody else has that same kind of experience."

One caregiver told me about a date with a guy who was also a caregiver. They hit it off, but with two caregiving schedules to manage, they never saw each other again. Another caregiver shared with our group her experience of going out with someone who also had an ill parent. She felt after one date he got attached too quickly because of their similar family situations while he didn't know much else about her; it made her uncomfortable. Other members chimed in they had also "felt suffocated" by those who seemed to be seeking a connection built on experiencing similar traumas.

Dr. Lisa raised the possibility that dating another caregiver may feed into overidentifying with your caregiver role. "If it works, it works. I can see all of the reasons why it could be safe and familiar and feel less threatening, because there's a point of reference. But I also can see how [if] everyone is running on low reserves then…who shows up and gives support to the other one?" She suggests asking yourself what it is you want from dating or a partner. "Every individual caregiver needs to ask themselves, do I need a partner that gets me out of this and can be a sole source of support for me? Or do I have enough room to also be a supportive co-caregiver to their parents or family member?"

Does Caregiving Impact the Partners We Choose?
There is finding a partner when you are already caregiving, and there is finding caregiving when you already have a partner. Either way, you hope you're partnered with someone who is on board. I've heard some people talk about the relationships caregiving broke, and others talk about the ones for which caregiving solidified their commitment to each other.

Whereas Kaci's current relationship began when she was already deep into caring for her mom, her previous relationship didn't have the benefit of the knowledge of what was to come. "We were together for five years. He went through a lot of that with me and I think I also was struggling with mental health stuff, especially that first year. I had a lot of resentment, started going back to therapy, was diagnosed with C-PTSD [complex PTSD]....That was tough, and then in the end...he left." Her current relationship began with caregiving already under her belt because she had a determination to get out there and figure out the logistics to make it work.

Debra has been caring for her mom since she was nineteen and believes that for the first few years a fear of judgment, for herself and her mom, subconsciously kept her from dating. Now she's married, but before their engagement Debra posted about their relationship: "The right partner will embrace you regardless and see the amazing strengths you possess as a caregiver. My mom's functioning really declined just a few months into my current relationship. I had to leave town abruptly and didn't see him for six weeks! But...I couldn't ask for a better partner. He has gone with me to Alzheimer's info sessions and an elder law attorney. He stepped up in ways I couldn't have imagined and I have to believe there are others out there just as good and loving."

Lea was dating someone in college when her mom required surgery for complications of Crohn's disease. The surgery resulted in its own major complications, so on weekends Lea drove from her dorm in Texas to care for her mom in Tennessee. On top of the two part-time jobs she held, time for her relationship was severely limited. "He knew the only way he was going to get to see me was he was going to have to go down [to Tennessee] with me and so he surprised me and came down one night. That was one of the moments that I had got up, I was kind of half asleep, and she had a [colostomy bag] leak....My boyfriend at the time, who is now my husband, was by my side at three o'clock in the morning cleaning out colostomy bags. This guy that I've only been with for, like, three months, he's there with my mom with her entire stomach hanging open, by my side just being there to support me."

After caregiving for my dad, I noticed how I refocused the qualities I look for in a partner. Predominantly, are they giving to others? Are they caring? I realized through my dad's illness and, ultimately, losing him that work is important to me, but the people you love are everything. I know firsthand what I am willing to devote to those close to me, that I put my money where my mouth is. I saw that this was a value shared with, probably inherited from, my family. It's a value that, before caring, I didn't truly realize the importance of. Or that it was instrumental. I know what I'm willing to give, so will this person offer the same to me? Are they there for their family? Inevitably, there will be more difficulties in life, so what choices do they make when confronted with hard realities? What and who are their priorities? Is this a value we share, because to me it's make or break.

WHEN IN A COMMITTED PARTNERSHIP

Alexandra's move from Thailand, where she lived and worked, to upstate New York to care for her mom uprooted her from her then-boyfriend, whose support she described as "angelic." Trying to salvage their partnership and to be present, her boyfriend moved back to Canada, where he was from, to be closer to Alex. The relationship was still long distance, but they were dedicated: after working long restaurant shifts, he would drive to spend Sunday and Monday with Alex before returning to work on Tuesday. "It was really brutal. And I went up a few times as well. But I just found that he was wonderful and he was so supportive and he was the dream, like to do all of that for me, but I couldn't go from this, like, caretaker role to then going back to like being a sexy, fun girlfriend. I couldn't connect the two and it really drove...I can't say *drove us apart*, because it was me, but it drove me apart from him."

In listening to Alex relay her experience of this previous relationship, what struck me was the two identities Alex felt she needed to uphold. I mentioned that, in light of everything she was doing for her mom, it sounded like a lot of pressure to put on herself to be that lighthearted girlfriend for him. "Absolutely. Yeah. I found it hard to connect. It was like I was dropping into this other life entirely. I found it hard to connect into the life I had before and the life I kind of have now."

From the outside, the pressure appeared to be self-generated. Alex's boyfriend had already moved across the world and taken a job he hated to be closer to her, so I had to think that if she didn't show up to visit him as the "sexy, fun girlfriend" but instead as the Alex who was there for her mom and was also spending the weekend in Canada to be with someone she loved, he would have accepted her. So, where did this pressure come from? I wondered whether the dissonance wasn't so much geographical but emotional, if the two personal worlds Alex lived in were so emotionally distant from each other that she didn't know how to marry them? She said:

Absolutely. I was living so much in the moments of having to go to the ER and the bad seizures and, you know, my mom crying when she couldn't... when she realized she had accidents. And I could never leave those moments entirely. So even when I was having my me-time and trying to keep my relationship alive or my career alive or all of these things, like, my mind was still in those worst moments. And I couldn't really leave them.

More than half (53.6 percent) of Millennials already caring for parents reported their significant others as very supportive.[5] Although this sounds like good news, and it is, caregiving can strain relationships, even those in early stages, despite a partner's support. The management of competing identities is difficult especially when, like Alex, you're haunted by disturbing images of a loved one in medical distress. These images can be difficult, or even feel impossible, to put aside. Especially when the anxiety of being away or an impending medical emergency constantly simmers in the background. Alex is not an outlier; this is something that I often hear from caregivers and that I experienced myself. It's not as easy as a change of outfit or location to switch into another mindset, to be present with your partner. Can we marry these two identities, or is this also an impossible task?

Kaci's current relationship also began long distance and, though she says people assumed it was difficult, she believes those three years were good for her. Caring for her mom is hard and the geographic distance allowed her some independence. Now with her boyfriend living nearby, Kaci has been able to strike a balance among the roles of caregiver, daughter, and girlfriend—but not without complications. Although she was up-front about her role as a caregiver when they began dating, she finds her boyfriend still doesn't fully understand the responsibility and why she has to be so physically present with her mom; she says it's the hardest part. "Sometimes we get in arguments where he's like, why can't you just leave her and come here? Like, you don't have to be in the house overnight. And I'm like, yes, I do. Like, legally I do. I can't just leave her for eight hours and then come back in the morning."

Whereas more than half said their partner was very supportive of their caregiving role, almost as many (43.5 percent of Millennials already caring for parents) reported parental care had caused arguments with their significant other.[6] Resentment about how much time is being given to the person being cared for and disagreements over such things as scheduling or spending on care or where the person needing care should live can cause rifts. Although it affects both of you, these topics may feel especially triggering when you are the caregiver and feel your partner doesn't understand the weight of responsibility or the added pull of it being your loved one. The stress of this decision-making can feel so intense, some Millennials reported fighting with their partner over care when they were still in the planning stages and not yet in the caregiver role.[7] Confronting choices like, *Do we both agree to live with the person who needs care?* can be a doozy on relationships at any age, particularly when you are younger and may have children in the house (or are yet to have a kid).

Not long after Rachel gave birth to a premature baby, her mom was diagnosed with the same debilitating disease her father had already died of years earlier. Having a baby while caring for her mom was exhausting, and she noticed the toll it took on her physical health. On top of it, she and her husband had different ideas when it came to caring for her mom. Rachel was able to move her mom closer to their family, but, with her mom's savings running out, more considerations on where she would live were to come. Rachel said her husband acknowledges the stress she's under and the toll caregiving has taken, but he won't help and doesn't want her mom to move in with them. His response adds to her emotional stress, which is already intense.

Debbie and her husband had been married for less than two years when it became clear her mom could no longer live alone. Debbie considered moving her mom in with her and her husband; she had seen other care-givers commit to this decision and thinks if both partners are on board, it could work. She weighed the effect her mom living with them would have on her marriage and decided assisted living was the best option. Although the decision was made to protect her marriage and avoid potential con-flict, she still feels guilt at times, despite the positive experience her mom has had living in a care facility.

The added stress of the situation can also intensify other issues in the relationship, even benign ones, and cause people to lose patience. One caregiver in her thirties said that, during the pandemic, she moved her mother in to live with her and her family; it caused all sorts of prob-lems. With her mom, who had cancer, and kids all under one roof, she was spread thin from addressing all of their needs. Emotional break-downs were common, as were fights with her husband. Still, she knew it was "the right thing" for the moment. (Her mom is now living inde-pendently again.)

Kaci's caregiving, particularly her mom's regular presence, has caused other conflicts in her relationships because she gets to hear her mom's unsolicited opinions on her boyfriends. "She's always disapproving, that's the other thing. Like no one's ever good enough....It's more of an issue [that] they take time away [from her], right? So there's some of that weird measurement stuff when you start caregiving, where it becomes this weird codependent thing, and so that's tough." This competition for Kaci's time that her mom expresses becomes even more heated when she doesn't like who Kaci is dating. "[She] and my current boyfriend are like oil and water together. I'm scared to leave them in a room together.... He's very strongly opinionated too and sometimes gets, I think, frustrated with the situation."

That's a love triangle I didn't expect: Kaci–Boyfriend–Kaci's Mom. There's the internal struggle we feel over giving our energy where it's needed, but now, when we do, like Kaci, we may also get to hear our family's unsolicited opinions on the regular. I was reminded of a time when, visiting my dad at his nursing home, I griped that my mom was setting me up on dates with total strangers she'd met on the street. (Sidenote: it's less scary than it sounds, she actually has a pretty good track record.) "Your mother wants to marry you off," my dad said, sitting in his wheelchair and loosening the laces on his sneakers so he could change his shoes. I watched carefully that he could but stood back to allow him to do it himself. "And so do I." Thanks for that. I asked Kaci how she coped.

"Therapy.... I always talk about how therapy has been really great for me as a caregiver and some people think that's weird, or they're like, 'Oh, I do music and exercise.' I'm like, that's cute, but I actually need someone to talk with me, work through these things with me." When her mom would piss her off complaining about her boyfriend, Kaci used to "throw in the white towel." Now, her therapist taught her to draw boundaries when it comes to her mom's unsolicited input. "I've gotten better about being able to say, 'I'm not having this conversation right now' or 'this conversation is not appropriate,' and being able to leave that there and not feel like I have to fix it."

Even when caregiving doesn't cause outright disagreements with your significant other, it can still affect the decisions you make together regarding your future. Will we need to move to be closer to family? Considering care expenses, can we afford a wedding? A house? Children?

"When people go into life-changing decisions out of alignment, it is a perfect breeding ground for resentment down the line...[or] for covert entitlement to check out," Dr. Lisa said. "Like, 'you made this decision, I didn't want to do it...I backed you in spite of myself, now I feel entitled to (fill in the blank).'" It's important to acknowledge that caregiving may fracture the vision you shared for your lives and the myriad feelings—from blame to regret and grief—that can be tied up in that. She recommends being proactive with a game plan to preserve privacy, peace, and finances, and to bring a therapist in for these tough conversations. "I always think it's useful to have a third-party position some of these questions that maybe we're blind to when we're in high emotional states or we're only seeing it through our lens. But I also think it depends on the couple. Some couples are really high-level communicators and can do it with low volatility, high compassion, high empathy. Some people can't, and I think if you can't...when opinions are out of alignment it can get volatile or spicy fast. Get in with someone [professional] quickly because the stakes are so high."

At the end of the day, Dr. Lisa said whether you're caregiving or not, it's important to stay attuned to the emotional needs of your significant other—and don't be afraid to ask for the same in return. "Part of what you sign up for is, 'I'm your person.' So I think it's fair game to [say], I would like you to be attuning to me." Also, caregivers should not forget about the needs of their partner. "I think it works both ways...the person who is the primary caregiver has to be sensitive to the fact that their time is being split in ways that weren't initially in the cards and what that means for themselves and for their partner."

ARE KIDS IN MY FUTURE?

I don't want to disparage the family we already have, but if you want it, there is an inclination to fantasize about the family you will inevitably grow for yourself. Who will my partner be? Partner or not, do I want kids? How many? When you're deep into caregiving, the question becomes: Will I ever have my own family?

When Michelle was in need of emotional support, at her breaking point in balancing her mom's care with her own career while living at home, she attended a group for working women caregivers. When she arrived, most of the women there were in their fifties. While in some ways she found support there, the disconnect she felt from women in a different stage of life put her in a panic. "The people in attendance were these moms. They were talking about their struggles raising their kids and then trying to caretake for their parents. And then there is this overwhelming feeling that I suddenly got, like, what if I never get to that? What if I never get to having my own family?" Her fear was palpable. Michelle had lived most of her life with her parents and had observed her own aunts and uncles care for her grandmother and then remain single. "They're all just living home together, siblings, and they're fine with that. But it's like, that's not what I want for myself in the future." She feels resentment toward the people who struggle with a family she would love to have but fears she never will, while still acknowledging their difficulties, too.

"Kids are always kind of at the back of our mind because I think before he got sick, it would have been a no-brainer," Casey told me. Since childhood, she'd always wanted to be a wife and mother, but her husband's chronic illness makes the added responsibility of children difficult to fathom. Still, he wants children. Casey wonders whether his understanding of the effort it takes to raise children is realistic. Familiar with the physical strain and the germs kids bring home, her mind turns over questions: Would a child's presence affect my husband's long-term health? . . . Could it make him permanently worse? . . . Could what he has be genetic?

> Now with his limitations, it's just a little bit more complicated. . . . I've gotten more accustomed to the idea of not having children even though it's very heartbreaking. But it's hard to balance what am I afraid to do, what do I think will be too much work and break me, versus how much joy could a kid bring? It's a really tough thing that we haven't figured out yet.

Casey questioning what may "break" her is a serious consideration. She already experienced a bout of panic attacks resulting from caregiving. Adding a child into the mix, whose daily life activities she would also likely be solely responsible for, is a massive consideration not only for her schedule but also for her mental health. This conversation was difficult for her; when she raised the idea of moving closer to extended family instead of growing her own, she stopped midsentence: "We might not have our own kids, but he's got two nieces and a nephew and so maybe that would be like our 'adopted children.' And so—sorry, I'm getting all choked up.... It's hard to lose the future you thought you'd have."

To better inform her thinking around the decision, Casey outsourced the question. She approached the various online support groups she's a member of (including Caregiver Collective) for practical insight on having children in light of a parent's chronic illness. She was surprised by the response. "I honestly expected everyone to say, if you have kids already, that's great. But if you don't have kids, don't have kids...it's going to be too much work. And so I was really interested to read kind of the more positive sides of things because I tend to think a lot more pessimistically since I would be the one doing most of the work. And so I think it opened my mind up a little bit more to: this would be doable. You just have to have the expectation that it's going to be a lot of work, but don't be opposed to having that joy in your life."

In our caregiver group, Beck was one of the people to respond to Casey's inquiry. Beck is forty-one and two years ago made the decision to have a baby with the platonic life partner he cares for, who is disabled and now showing signs of dementia. "A while back an older caregiver friend of mine looked me in the eye and said, 'Beck, none of my dreams came true.' In that moment I vowed to make my one big dream come true.... The pressure and workload of caring for a baby and a senior scares me every single day, but words can't describe the joy of this sweetest dream coming true."

Beck imagines it to be similar to being a single parent of two. He handles all the diaper and clothing changes, takes his son to day care. "It's more work than I could have ever imagined. However, my partner can sit and hold the baby and give bottles and love and laughter and ride him around on her mobility scooter and they have the sweetest relationship."

So how does Beck do it, really? He's hired a professional in-home care-giver to work forty hours a week so it's "doable." Unable to afford the expense on his own, they held a GoFundMe campaign to finance the help.

When it comes to giving advice, Beck doesn't sugarcoat: "I'm the one who wanted a baby so damn bad, so I'm glad we did it and I don't regret it. If you are not the one [who] one hundred percent wants this, then I'd say it'll be too much. But if you one hundred percent want it, then it's doable. Because once you do it, you have to do it, if that makes sense.... I've caregived for seventeen years straight and it's been an unimaginable amount of work, and I even had custody of a godson on and off for many years, but nothing prepared me for the amount of work for basically solo caregiving for a newborn/baby/toddler."

Kaci's caregiving experience also cemented her decision regarding future children. "I think, for me, kids: definitely no. I don't want them anymore." She feels that she exchanged the freedom of her younger years, to live abroad and to make free choices, for her mom's needs. Later in life, when she is no longer needed as her mom's caregiver, she wants to make up for lost time. "I want to be able to travel someday and I think if I have children that would make it really difficult because I [didn't] get to have those experiences in my twenties."

WHO WILL CARE FOR US?

One unpartnered caregiver in my group who cares for both parents with dementia was filling out her own medical forms and realized she didn't know who to list as next of kin. It's a logistical problem, sure: If you've been in a car accident, let's say, who should the hospital call? But the underlying issue is: When I'm in need, who's there to care for me?

We know how each of our family units look today. But what will our families look like decades down the line? When we're older and in need of care, who will help us?

Of Millennials with children, more than half said they expected their kids to take care of them one day.[8] That sounds nice in the hypothetical, but as a representative of those caring now, we know what a responsibility that job is—particularly when you're the only one to take on the role. About 20 percent of households with children today are one-child families;[9] only-child families are the fastest-growing family unit in the United States.[10] Almost half of LGBTQ+ Millennials are actively planning to grow their families, just slightly less than non-LGBTQ+ Millennials (which is a much narrower gap than for previous generations).[11] Although the pandemic did result in a small baby bump, particularly in women ages thirty to thirty-four (most likely because they were working from home), it remains likely that families with Millennial parents will remain small.[12]

AND FOR THOSE WITHOUT KIDS, THEN WHAT? THE EMOTIONAL WEIGHT of whether or not you partner up or have children has very practical and economic implications. No one wants to be alone. Luckily, we are a generation whose idea of family structure has evolved into something more fluid. In an article for *Vox*, Laura St. James writes about the rise and current state of the chosen family, mostly associated with the queer community:

> *The prevalence of traumatic backgrounds within queer spaces, however, makes them uniquely well-suited to discussing and processing those backgrounds. And the more that a collective awareness of how trauma operates moves through into the American mainstream, the more that queer ideas about chosen family also move into the mainstream. As queer people are being granted greater legal protections, so long as our family structures replicate the nuclear family structure, it follows that cishet [cisgender, heterosexual] people are adopting more ideas about how family might consist of the friends you are especially close to, not just your family of origin (see: the rise of Friendsgiving).[13]*

We already see the existence of chosen families in caregiving today. But what about when we're still healthy and thinking toward the future? Recently, my IG Reels were flooded with the story of seven female friends in China who decided to "Golden Girls" it, according to the *New York Post*.[14] They collectively bought and renovated a house where they plan to retire together later in life. This new vision of families and the idea of creating spaces in which they can operate has been a fun conversation topic for a while now—even the actual Golden Girls were onto each other. We are cognizant of our desire to be taken care of and by the people in our lives we love, no matter how untraditionally those relationships evolve later in life.

CHAPTER 7

IN SICKNESS AND IN HEALTH: CARING FOR YOUR SIGNIFICANT OTHER

I struggle with my identity as a girlfriend a lot, right? Because he's just so fatigued that he can't be affectionate as much, and so oftentimes I feel like a mom because I'm like, "Here's your medicine." Or I feel like a nurse or a house-keeper because the chores are just so unequally divided now that I'm having to do things for a house that isn't mine. It just feels a little strange.

—Casey, 35

CASEY DESCRIBES HER PARTNER BEFORE HIS ILLNESS AS REALLY OUTGO-ing, caring, warm, and charismatic, with a booming voice and a laugh heard "before you even walk in." She respects his intelligence (he holds a PhD in nuclear engineering) and they had fun together. Both "pretty nerdy" (her words), before he got sick one of their favorite things to do was make their own cosplay costumes and go to Comic Cons. She knows that unless there's a significant change to his health, it's something they'll never do together again.

Caregiving for a spouse or partner is often overlooked when we think about family care at our age, when partners are most likely not elderly. These partnerships may be a lot newer; at a younger age, it's much less likely you've already been together for decades. When I discuss these care scenarios with someone new to the idea, more than once I've been met with, *I wouldn't do it.* The thought of taking on this hefty role seems an unnecessary hardship to some, so why put yourself through it? Most likely, these people have not been in the position themselves. They aren't taking into account how meeting the right person can feel like a fortuitous lightning strike. This person isn't replaceable to you; the partnership you've built includes shared history, commitment, and devotion. There can still be times of joy.

That said, have I heard of relationships ending because of unexpected illness or disability? Yes. Instances exist where one person did not want to commit to a relationship that included care of another at this level, or the afflicted partner did not want to put another person in that position. Like many family and care choices, we can't judge from the outside but only trust what happens is for the best. And: it's none of our business.

Other times, the couple stays together, but care creates a tension they find difficult to overcome. One member of the Collective expressed they were "losing empathy and kindness" for their partner, who, they felt, didn't help out or care for themselves in ways they were still able to. The caregiving partner felt unconsidered and that they were being taken for granted. Although they didn't express wanting to break up, they did question how much longer they could go on in that situation.

For those who stay committed, walking away may feel unthinkable, but there is no denying that the nature of the relationship changes; the balance of reciprocity is thrown off when unexpected chronic or fatal illness dictates days and lifestyle. Depending on the diagnosis, dependency and its impact on the relationship can vary.

With his illness, Casey's partner is physically unable to care for himself. His brain fog and fatigue are so bad that the exertion of sending a single work email "knocks him on his butt." They were still dating when Casey moved into his apartment to care for him around the clock. At the time, she told me their conversations mostly revolved around his needs, from scheduling doctor appointments to what he could eat that day. She estimates caregiving comprises about 90 percent of their relationship. Because he is severely immunocompromised, she doesn't receive any outside help. They are happily married now, and Casey remains optimistic and upbeat, but she also referred to caregiving as a "life-altering ultra-exhausting grieving process of no longer having my own life."

Caregivers can find, or at least imagine and attempt, an outlet in social connections and romantic relationships. Hanging out with peers who offer a reprieve can help connect you to your own life again. But, for Casey, caring for her partner means her romantic relationship is irreversibly changed. Casey makes sure they do activities together as a couple, though it's a big adjustment. "Finding new fun things to do together that are extremely low energy has been challenging. Before the pandemic, we were just really social and hung out with a lot of people from church and had a lot of holiday and birthday parties together. Now everything is over Zoom [because of his illness], but even that takes up all of his energy. So we just have to be very careful about what our social life looks like."

Casey described her relationship as "super supportive of each other." They are open about discussing their problems, but he wears out so quickly now that sometimes he'll tell her he's not up for it and the talk will be tabled for a couple of weeks. But when it comes to the challenges of caregiving, Casey isn't as open. So many people I spoke with who didn't have partners hoped they could find someone to support them through their caregiving. Some caregivers expressed that they felt extra supported when their partners not only observed their care work but jumped in to help. I wondered about Casey and her husband's relationship, whether she was open with him about her feelings around care.

"If I let him know just super honestly how I'm struggling, then he'll just wear out immediately because he's worried [that] he's stressed me out, that he's putting me in a situation where I'm burdened with a lot of things, and so I usually don't tell him all of the … struggles or the things that I'm going through just because I want him to be okay." It's a pretty big thing not to share with your partner, but Casey says her support system is strong. When it comes to these particular stresses and worries, she turns to her mom, whom she calls her best friend, as well as friends she knows she can vent to and our caregiver support group.

ADJUSTING MARRIAGE EXPECTATIONS

Any care relationship requires balancing ideals with realities and abilities and adjusting expectations. When you are caring for the person you are in a romantic relationship with, these adjustments can take on a different tenor: they can affect your engagement and what your wedding is like or if you decide to have one at all.

"Maybe it just needs to be he and I on the sofa with a pastor," Casey told me about her wedding planning at the time. Although her dream was to have a large in-person wedding surrounded by family and friends, she was realistic. What kind of wedding ceremony was plausible without damaging her fiancé's health—possibly for the rest of his life? She had already witnessed how scouting venues and buying wedding outfits had led to a "really bad crash." "Maybe we could stream something instead of having people there in person, which is just a whole new set of grief to deal with. Because I think we just both had this idea of a wedding as a chance to have all of your friends there...everyone coming together and having a fun little party to support each other. And so not having that, I think, would be a heartbreak. But we've got our outfits. We're gonna look good."

It can be heartbreaking to hear someone correlate their upcoming wedding with grief, but caregiving at our age has the capacity to dramatically change meaningful rites of passage into something other than expected or hoped for. (That's not to say they can't still be great; Casey and her fiancé pulled off a wedding that accommodated their needs, which she called "a monumental task," and it was "even more beautiful than we ever imagined!")

Some people caring for partners had to adjust their expectations for marriage in other ways, possibly shelving it entirely—solely because of their care role. Shortly after Zoe became engaged, her fiancé was diagnosed with a terminal cancer. Quickly, his ability to move around on his own and take care of himself became difficult, and Zoe quit her job to become his full-time caregiver. In light of his illness, they decided to get married as soon as possible...until they learned spouses were not eligible to be paid by the state as caregivers. She turned to the Collective for advice: other members chimed in with stories of also being ineligible for caregiver pay as a spouse and the need to hire an eldercare attorney to help navigate your rights within the system. It shone a light on what one member referred to as "a marriage penalty" for those on disability. The most uplifting suggestions: to have a wedding ceremony anyway, exchange rings, but as a religious or spiritual event and not a legal marriage.

WHEN YOUR SPOUSE FEELS MORE LIKE YOUR ROOMMATE

Lizzie's husband contracted COVID on Father's Day weekend—as she calls it, "the horrible irony." When Lizzie and I spoke, it had been over a year since he'd developed symptoms and in that time they'd progressed horribly. Lizzie keeps a spreadsheet of symptoms to share with doctors: chest palpitations and pressure, migraines, persistent insomnia that results in brain fog and debilitating fatigue and exhaustion. It had forced him to take medical leave from work. Sensitive to sound and unable to function, her husband is up most of the night; they now keep separate bedrooms.

I noticed Lizzie didn't spend much time telling me about her relationship with her husband "before." "He was an awesome person," she told me. Instead, she is very much focused on her to-do list, which is dominated by their two small children (ages two and four), and balancing their needs with her career. Lizzie has begun to think of herself as a single mom. Like any overwhelmed parent, her focus squarely prioritizes her kids. As her husband's condition has worsened, she's also taken on more of his care (researching his condition and long COVID medical programs, scheduling and taking him to doctor appointments, etc.) as well as the household responsibilities he used to manage.

I asked what their relationship is like now. Lizzie was very matter-of-fact: "I don't want to say it's gone. But it's roommates." She expressed guilt about having these thoughts, knowing at times he is still available to her emotionally; it's something she sometimes forgets:

I have now shifted to usually seeing him as someone that I need to care for, not a partner. He still actually—I have breakdowns and he is great....He can provide some emotional support. I just usually feel bad when I kind of unload because I'm always like, I complain about me being tired. You haven't slept in a year.

When you boil it down, Lizzie was explaining the loss of her partner. He is still physically present but unable to maintain the relationship they had. It felt obtuse to ask how that made her feel, but...how did she feel? Questions that required her to consider her emotions, not the logistical help she needed, took Lizzie an extra minute to answer. "I haven't even ever really processed it because I don't have time. Like I kind of...I mean, [I feel] sad, for sure."

Referring to a partner you care for as a "roommate" is something I've heard a few times in my caregiving group. Dr. Lisa recommends having an honest conversation with your partner about how care has changed your relationship. Although she calls this "a partner activity," she acknowledges the conversation can be incredibly difficult. "There is a huge elephant in the room that I think people in those dynamics do not confront. Because it's hard, because there's no answer, there's no resolve, right? Because it's really just acknowledgment for acknowledgment's sake. And yet in acknowledgment for acknowledgment's sake is a lot of healing or a lot of catharsis, or it creates, again, a little bit of that sense of 'you're still my person who's able to see me.'" She suggests it may be helpful to have a therapist or other third party there to facilitate.

INTIMACY

"How do you make sure your needs are being met while also respecting the limited range of what your partner is (or isn't) able to give you?" one caregiver asked. "I'm struggling with this and don't know how to continue this relationship without jeopardizing my body image and sexual needs. I feel so bad for even bringing the conversation up, but the rejection I experience over and over again is really damaging my self-esteem and causing me to resent the relationship."

How physical intimacy is navigated with each other, if at all, is another consideration when couples face the changed physical abilities of one partner. Some caregivers choose to employ what Dr. Lisa referred to as a "very fabulous masturbation habit" to meet their own needs; for others, the loss of sexual intimacy is not a high priority, so they elect acceptance. For caregivers for whom it is a high priority, the shift in sexual intimacy with their partner leads to redefining the terms of their relationship. While caring for his wife, one caregiver shared how the years-long lack of sexual intimacy affected him psychologically: he "disassociated" from his body. The couple made the "hard choice" to open their relationship, but he saw a very positive effect from reconnecting with this part of his identity. Couples may not anticipate turning to ethical nonmonogamy or polyamory, but some feel it's the only option to remain together when one provides care for the other.

"From a sexual standpoint, I think different people manage in different ways," Dr. Lisa said. "Some people take someone on the side, and people will morally judge that or they won't. I think that depends on where you stand in it." She advises caregivers to evaluate their needs and the priority of those needs in their life and don't limit it to just the physical:

> *There's emotional intimacy, social intimacy, sexual, recreational, intellectual. Depending on where the need falls for you, if it is a high-level need, it is going to have to be serviced somehow. If emotional intimacy is of high importance to you, and it is no longer available in your primary romantic relationship, I think the question you ask yourself is, "Where do I now get this need met? Does that mean I get it met in an emotional affair?"... [Or] "I recognize that romantic emotional intimacy is not going to be part of my world anymore, but can I find very rich emotional intimacy in friendship?" Certainly, I think you need to ask yourself where your boundaries are.*

DESPITE BEING CONSUMED WITH HER KIDS, LIZZIE DOESN'T OVERLOOK the need for physical intimacy—for both her and her husband:

> I feel like we need to try and watch a movie or snuggle on the couch or have some kind of physical touch because I feel like both of us need that. I'm kind of aware of that. But I just, I feel like I don't even have time to be sad about it. I'm sure it's there underneath the surface—I'm, like, tearing up now. I'm usually like, go, go, go. Gotta get something done.

"Go, go, go" is something she's been doing for a while. The couple had been in the throes of a new baby's first year (what she called "survival mode") and were finally able to get the kids into post-lockdown day care when her husband got sick. Spending quality time together as a couple has been a long time coming; even sick, he comes in second to the kids for claims on Lizzie's attention. "I would like him to know that I still care about him and I'm here for him, but he always tells me the kids come first and I sort of feel like the kids come first too. They can't do anything on their own yet. I'm usually depleted by the time I'm done being their everything. But I look at him and I'm like, *Oh my God.*"

They've thought of trying to get away for a few days without the kids, just the two of them. An upcoming wedding in Rhode Island could be the perfect opportunity; even if he doesn't attend the event, they can spend quality time together away. "I can't really leave him without anything emotionally," she told me. "And then I know it helps me, too."

CHAPTER 8

THE SANDWICH GENERATION GIVES RISE TO THE MULTIGENERATIONAL CAREGIVER

I keep having this fear that if he doesn't go back to work, that I'm the sole care-taker and the sole breadwinner. And that's a lot. To be frank, I don't even like saying this out loud, but I feel like, for your book, it's like, "Oh, if you passed away, I'd be in the same scenario but with survivors' benefits. But you're here, which means I need to take care of you and them on maybe only my salary." Which is terrifying.

—Lizzie, 34

WITHOUT HER HUSBAND AS A HANDS-ON PARTNER, LIZZIE'S HAD TO take on solo parenting of their two small children, and the lapse of support has left her fearful of the future—not to mention exhausted in the day-to-day. She's running the household and taking care of all three while maintaining her career in (get this) healthcare consulting. There are pick-ups and drop-offs to day care, calls to doctor offices, meals to be cooked and fed, and a full workday. She has no time to be sick herself; a recent curbside pickup from Target for a simple box of Cheerios was postponed for days because she had the stomach flu.

It didn't start this way. When Lizzie's husband first developed COVID and his symptoms were milder, he was able to continue working. Liz-zie, meanwhile, took on being a full-time parent—while also work-ing her actual full-time job remotely from home. The couple expected his condition to improve as a normal case would; instead, in subsequent weeks and months his health worsened.

In the beginning, he could handle his own medical care. Eventually, as symptoms progressed and he was granted medical leave from his job, even calling doctors became difficult for him... and, as people with chronic illness in the United States know, when dealing with doctors and insurance companies, a lot of calls need to be made to get anywhere. "He couldn't do it. You'd have to get on hold and wait forever to talk to someone to schedule an appointment and if you are (a) depressed and (b) don't feel well, you don't have the time for that."

Lizzie took on scheduling and escorting him to doctor appointments, has access to his medical chart, and takes notes in medical appointments. She keeps a spreadsheet to track symptoms and treatments they've tried and records the results. Within the household, she noticed lapses in bill payments he was responsible for so transitioned household contracts to her name so that she could handle the family's financial management herself.

Crunched in the middle of child-rearing and being caregiver to her husband, Lizzie isn't quite the sandwich generation we grew up hearing about—simultaneously caring for small kids and elderly parents. Instead, Lizzie is a multigenerational caregiver.[1] Although there are many possible combinations, multigenerational caregiving can include raising kids while also providing care for a partner, a sibling, a close friend... or, yes, an ailing senior family member. Or maybe children aren't part of the equation and you're caring for two adults of different generations, such as a spouse and a parent. This phenomenon isn't new, but it is a trend that's on the rise—particularly in our generation. Just over half of multigenerational caregivers with a child at home under the age of eighteen are between the ages of thirty and forty-four years (another 15 percent are eighteen to twenty-nine).[2] In other words, the majority of people who are raising a dependent child while also providing care to another family member (of any age) are Millennials or in Gen Z.

Caring for her husband and lacking his physical support have put pressure on Lizzie to be more available to her children. She relies on her seventy-year-old mom to fill in where she struggles; Lizzie doesn't know how she would manage without her mother's help. "She will come over and help with the kids almost any time I ask, she's my backup. I'm terrified for the day that that changes because I still rely on my mom for a lot of help to be my support person. So the day that I might have to be in charge of her care is just currently terrifying."

Her mom is the only person, aside from Lizzie's therapist, who knows the family's situation and difficulties. Lizzie has a couple of friends she talks to for emotional support but holds back from confiding fully because she worries her honesty could sound like she's bad-mouthing her husband. If she didn't have her mom nearby, she'd look into local teenagers to babysit but can't imagine incurring that cost regularly in addition to the kids' day care. She fears her husband won't be physically able to resume work after his medical leave and they'll become a single-income family of four.

ECONOMIC FALLOUT

Economic insecurity is a valid fear for a lot of families in the United States. Just before the pandemic, most Millennial households (66 percent) with a married couple and a child under the age of eighteen operated with the incomes of both parents.[3] The pandemic exacerbated any financial stretch and created new hardships, with women leaving the workforce in record numbers to shift duties to full-time childcare. In fact, for Lizzie's family, it was the need to go back to work when offices reopened that, ultimately, resulted in her husband getting COVID: when adult vaccines became available, Lizzie and her husband chose to resume their prepandemic work schedules; one of their kids contracted COVID-19 at day care.

Multigenerational caregivers in general (meaning with small kids or not) may be at the highest risk of negative repercussions of caregiving (financial strain, exiting the workforce, emotional stress, etc.) because of the cumulative effects of a "caregiving squeeze," being torn between caring for multiple family members with differing needs.[4] For a young family like Lizzie's in which a spouse is being cared for, the period of care may be significantly longer than when caring for someone elderly. The financial stress Lizzie fears is striking at an age of expected earning and savings potential and of "human capital accumulation" (building social relationships); the gamut of negative repercussions can interfere and have a longer time to accumulate.[5]

EMOTIONAL FALLOUT

A study by New York Life shows that, as a result of the pandemic, those caring for an aging relative and children reported less time spent per week on rest and relaxation, sleeping, physical exercise, quality time with loved ones, preparing and eating healthy meals, and caring for their own physical, mental, and emotional well-being.[6] Caregivers may grab at time to decompress whenever they can. One woman cares for her father-in-law, who suffers from a host of serious diagnoses, as well as for her intellectually disabled nephew. She also has her own kids, ranging in age from early elementary to high school age. She says her only happy place is Dunkin' Donuts and a quick drive to a home goods store.

Other multigen caregivers who wound up cohabitating with ailing loved ones describe the stress of having them under the same roof as their kids. Another caregiver in her thirties moved her family in with a grandmother who has dementia. She described her exhaustion dealing with two small children and a senior woman who has cognitive decline and strong opinions. She's frustrated other family doesn't help...even her dog keeps running away. *Even the dog*...it's like a country music song for our generation.

We also have to take into account those of us who care long distance. One caregiver said they had to leave their toddler and husband at home to care for their parent who had cancer—on the opposite coast. They were separated for months, an experience, they said, "almost broke me."

When caregiving balanced with parenting comes up in Caregiver Collective, the overwhelming sentiment is how difficult it is to be a caregiver to someone who is ailing but put it aside to parent the kids who still need you. The kids may be too young to understand or old enough to see what's going on and need extra emotional cushioning to comprehend and process it. Research shows Millennial parents prioritize their children's needs in general, but we can't deny the toll that takes—for any parent, but particularly caregivers whose lives are also clouded by a loved one's debilitated health.[7] Jayne is the mom of two small boys and unexpectedly lost her father shortly before taking on the care of her grandmother. "Taking on your children's daily needs also doesn't allow you the time to sit in your own sadness too long. That's good and bad. Keeping busy helped distract me, but I didn't process all that happened too well."

When it comes to managing the emotional aspect of how Lizzie's family has changed with her husband's illness, Lizzie focuses on her role as parent and on her children's adjustment. She doesn't discuss her own emotions surrounding her husband's long COVID with many people but does inform her kids' school and other parents to make sure the kids are supported. "I want people to know that my kids are going through something and [to] make sure they're okay."

In fact, Lizzie has a hard time even identifying as a caregiver; she thinks of herself primarily as an exhausted parent. When Lizzie told me that she didn't know if her problems were relevant to a book on family caregiving, my response was: "Are you kidding?" So much of the family story Lizzie shared boils down to: *How do I balance the life that I set up for myself before caregiving with the care necessary now?*

When many care needs tug at you, there's an instinct to give everything to care because you feel you have to, but Dr. Lisa warns it also may be a way to preoccupy yourself to avoid your own heavy feelings:

Make sure that you don't stay in such high perpetual motion... or that you don't forgo every need that you have at such a high level that you lose yourself, such that you either don't know who you are or you can't catch your breath. Because that's when I think you decompensate, and then if the caregiver goes down, the whole system falls.

When it comes to balancing the needs of multiple family members and surviving, Dr. Lisa said the "single healthiest thing" a caregiver can do is to make time for themselves. "I also recognize in that statement, anyone who is a caregiver probably wants to send me to go fuck myself." That said, breathing room is a critical resource and necessary inclusion. Dr. Lisa also recommends taking inventory of your needs: recognizing how you function and what you require. This isn't limited to logistical needs, like a babysitter who can pinch hit, but includes inventorying what you need to fill your own tank, like having a chatty dialogue with a friend. Ask yourself: *What are my needs this day, this week, this month? Are they being met? Who can help meet those needs, and am I outsourcing fairly?*

LIZZIE HAS NEW HOPE FOR HER HUSBAND'S RECOVERY NOW THAT HE'S been admitted to a long COVID program, but she knows things remain uncertain. Until then, managing the needs of her family remains in the crosshairs. When it comes to making time for herself, she admits that she's often reluctant to ask anyone to watch her kids because she feels guilty but knows it's something she needs to overcome. "I'm trying to get better at proactively asking for help," she said.

CHAPTER 9

MAINTAINING FRIENDSHIPS

IN THE WEEKS AFTER MY FATHER DIED, I SAW ONLY MY CLOSEST CHILD-hood friends, the people who had known me and my family the longest. They would come to my neighborhood and we'd do something simple, a walk or swinging in an empty playground; they knew I wasn't capable of much but needed comfort and distraction. One afternoon, Laura and I were walking uptown; she says we went to a museum, but I only remember the sidewalks with her by my side. In the only moment of that day I can recall, I was in the midst of crying. I didn't hide it, the impulse was unavoidable and unstoppable; the past few years were escaping through my tear ducts and it would be a lengthy process whose timeline I had no say in. My emotions swung regularly; I told Laura I was feeling rises of anger that I couldn't explain. She stopped in her tracks, looked at me, and offered soberly: "If you want, you can punch me in the face."

She really meant it, that I could see. It caught me off guard. I think I even laughed. *Wow,* I thought in amazement, *that's real friendship.* (I didn't take her up on the offer.)

This was years before Laura's father was diagnosed with dementia; she was unaware of what was down the road for her own family. She didn't yet know firsthand what being a caregiver to a dad you love so much, what losing him, felt like—or that she ever would. All she knew was that I was hurting.

I was, and am still, so grateful to the friends who showed up for me then. I had asked and they had arrived, no questions asked and no concessions requested. They were just there. I see now that Laura, or any of those friends, coming to spend an afternoon with me required bravery. You are showing up for someone who is in a bad place, you are offering to step into their world beside them, and you probably don't know what to do or say or expect. It can be scary.

Whereas bereavement was my big kahuna of grief, caregivers are experiencing various levels of loss and trauma the entire time they're managing everything that goes with the illness or aging of someone they love. Truthfully, when I was going through it, I really didn't let my friends in on much of what I was feeling or experiencing. I used time with them as a reprieve, a night or a lunch away from thinking about it all, to feel like everything was "normal." To convince myself it still was.

The friends I did let peek behind the curtain cared. They offered what they knew how and what I would allow. What I have seen more clearly since my caregiving experience is that it's important to have friends, or one friend, who will see you—really see you—and acknowledge what you are going through in a way that feels genuine. That requires you to open up. It's a life lesson I now won't compromise with myself on, but it's easier said than done, particularly if this is the first time you are making yourself vulnerable in this way. By *vulnerable* I mean: admitting you need real help. When you become a caregiver at a young age, your friends most likely have no experience with what you're living; it can be hard to grasp the magnitude of it from the outside. Your friendships may even become strained as the life you are living, the emotions you are experiencing, become further disconnected from what others are experiencing.

WHEN THERE'S A DISCONNECT

Amongst my mom's group of friends, there were so many people who were able and dying to help out. They were very close with her and they're of the

age where they may be taking care of their parents, so they actually have
some sense of what you need and how they can help. Whereas I felt like my
friends had no idea how to help...there were very few of them that could in
any way begin to wrap their heads around what was going on.

Alexandra wasn't even thirty when her mom was diagnosed with
glioblastoma and Alex moved back in to care for her. Brain cancer is a
diagnosis that requires heavy subsequent care: soon after, her mom was
paralyzed and required help with everything from daily life activities
to medical treatments. Alex was entering a familiar home that quickly
became a foreign world. Very soon, their communication was compromised; Alex was losing her mother and witnessing it day by day. It was
happening faster than she knew to expect. There were not many people
she knew her age, if any, who could relate to the intensity of those emotions, to the physical care required.

After the diagnosis, Alex had moved quickly from her home in Thailand to her mom's house in upstate New York, leaving her group of friends
and boyfriend behind. She put her involvement in planned projects for her
new business on hold and backed out of being a bridesmaid in a friend's
wedding because it coincided with her mom beginning radiation. She went
from being the center of a social circle to a new reality that was isolating,
that many of her friends couldn't relate to, and that she was unprepared for:

There's just so much so quickly that you give up, which almost maybe is like
a good thing because it just gets you. It breaks you really quick. You're like,
"Okay, my life for this short chapter is over." It was like trial by fire.

So much of Alex's life was consumed by cancer and care, she barely had
an opportunity to shower, never mind connect with friends. When she
did, the stark difference between the "normal" lives they were living—so
similar to her own life "before"—and the life she had at home with her
mom and stepdad, the harsh light of the world she used to inhabit, was
jarring and underscored her social disconnect.

Michelle's experience was more progressive and not quite the same trial by fire, but care also removed her from the normal social life of a woman in her twenties or thirties: "When you're not doing stuff for your loved one or for the home, then you're just straight up tired.... You just want to spend that time cocooning...until you have to take on the rest of the week." When she did have plans, she often had to cancel last minute because her mom wasn't feeling well and Michelle wouldn't leave her home alone. There's only so many times you can back out last minute, she said, before your friends stop inviting you altogether. Eventually, it was like she became "out of sight, out of mind."

I remember one caregiver, a woman in her early thirties, saying she dreaded summer because she knew everyone would be out at barbecues that she was never able to go to because she was caring at home for both parents. It went beyond FOMO—fear of missing out—to resentment. There's a mental health toll of not connecting socially, but you can also lose touch with the people important to you, the activities or events that define a particular time in your life.

Without that quality time with friends and sharing in experiences together, Michelle found she began to relate to them less. The social isolation only compounded the isolation the experience of caregiving had already made her feel.

There's another big reason Michelle felt isolated from her friends: there was an unspoken rule in her household not to share information about her mom's illness with anyone, even extended family. Michelle was left to process all this alone; she didn't dare ask anyone for help or share her experiences and emotions. As her mom's illness progressed, Michelle hit a breaking point and needed to talk to someone.

"I was just like, 'Okay, you know what? Whatever, I can trust my friend. It's fine.' So I started with the inner circle and then just organically I started to tell more people. And then I think there are times, though, when I felt like I shared it with certain colleagues or friends and then maybe overshare[d], like starting to become a bit of a Debbie Downer, and I could feel them kind of pull back." This feeling of being a Debbie Downer comes up a lot among people our age dealing with family illness. We've learned, either explicitly or implicitly, that disease and chronic illness are a negative talking point. Not only that, we're discussing it in intimate terms of how it is impacting our family directly; it's easy to see why we think others would think it's depressing: it can depress *us*. And if no one we know has experienced this, what can they possibly say? If their reaction doesn't match the gravity of what we're feeling, or is out of touch, it can be disappointing or hurtful. When caregivers reveal what they are feeling to a friend and are met with a reaction that they feel is dismissive, they clam up. In turn, sometimes when friends don't know what to say or they feel totally out of their depth, they also stop asking and can distance themselves. Caregivers tell me they feel "forgotten about."

That disconnect goes both ways: our friends can also feel like we don't understand what the hell is going on with them. When your time and energy is sucked up by care, you're often less available to support your friends when they need it. Your mind may be someplace else; and I'll be honest, in comparison to a chronic illness or terminal disease— truthfully—their problems may sound like bullshit. I remember going out with friends one night to get my mind off things, to try to recalibrate my nervous system by just having fun. My close friend at the time filled me in on the relationship goings-on of someone we both knew. For them, it was monumental and dramatic; I thought: *What in the hell am I listening to this for? These problems are vapid and ridiculous.* I actually felt angry that someone wasted their time on such frivolity; but, as Ron shared with me, what he at the time viewed as other people's frivolous problems he now sees were typical of-age issues and conversations. And, I think, he's right. When you're in the midst of it, though, and on such a separate plane of thought, your own lack of empathy can be hard to see.

The disappointing and sad truth is that some people lose friends because of caregiving; whether because of this disconnect or because how (or if) someone shows up reveals something about them you didn't otherwise see. Lizzie, whose husband has long COVID, talks openly about her family situation with her therapist, but not with her friends; they'd offer unsolicited advice when what she needs is support. Those who did offer help often didn't follow through; she began viewing their offers as empty platitudes. She found opening up to people in her life left her frustrated to the point that she stopped reaching out for help:

> *I have a couple of people who are very well meaning, but one was like, "What do you need?" and I said, "It was just really nice to go over to your house for dinner sometimes and not have to cook." And they say, "Oh, you're welcome anytime," but don't invite me. I have to call them and then sometimes when I've called them, it's like, "Oh, we're actually not going to do it this weekend." Like, I'm not gonna keep calling you.*

Another person in her life offered backup childcare, but when Lizzie called to take her up on it, the woman told her she couldn't do it. Asking for help is not easy. Lizzie mentioned multiple times that she is wracked with guilt asking favors to care for her kids since her husband became ill; having those cries for help go unheard or unheeded feels even worse. I've experienced this too: good friends I confided in when a family member was ill told me they would be there for me, and then weren't. I've learned, if the friendship feels worth it, to directly address this. In one instance, the friend apologized; she told me she thought I was receiving support from my closer friends and didn't know I needed her, too. Another friend grew defensive and, though he said he'd try to better support me, never mentioned what I was going through again. My grief was met with avoidance. I felt like he cared more that he was saying the right thing, but when it came down to it, he—most likely—didn't know how to handle it so ignored the topic entirely. It was probably emotional immaturity, but I judged him for it. Our friendship never returned to what it was before and ultimately ended. I didn't trust him as I once did.

HOW YOU CAN CONNECT WITH FRIENDS

After my father died, I remember my aunt telling me, "Your friends *want* to be there for you." I hadn't before thought about how my need for support would feel from their perspective. When I felt guilty for being the Debbie Downer, seeming needy, and knew the guilt was keeping me emotionally isolated, my therapist asked, "What if the shoe was on the other foot and it was your friend coming to you? Would you be annoyed or wish they hadn't?" Of course not. Although supporting you may not always be easy for your friends, I believe they will find it manageable. Your real friends are willing to handle it. If they don't know how, they will at least try in a way you can feel.

After this conversation with my aunt, I was back in Los Angeles and tried to resume my normal life. Grief after death is another form of imposter syndrome: despite the heavy cloud of emotions circling above, you push yourself through the motions of a regular day until it does, actually, start to feel normal again. I made plans to catch up with my friend Leo. He's not one of my closest friends; he didn't know what I had just been through. I pulled together a normal Jenn outfit as best I could and went to meet him at the spot he'd chosen near our apartments. My energy low, I felt a bit disconnected from my surroundings. After our hellos I told him, "I'm sorry, I'm not fully myself lately." I gave him the brief rundown that my father had died. I was teary just saying the words. I told him, "I feel badly that I'm not the person you were expecting to meet."

Leo took off the wooden bead bracelet he wore around his wrist and put it on mine. He'd gotten it from a guru, he said (at least that's my memory; in my mind it's the Dalai Lama, but he probably said he bought it at the Bali airport), and told me: "Everything you are right now is enough." He had given me permission to be genuine with him, to not put on a show. It told me that I still held value for him, even at my lowest. Almost ten years later, it's a mantra I still use; when I'm feeling depleted, I put on the bracelet as a physical reminder—of the message and of the friendship I received when I needed it.

By the time I went through a serious hospital experience with my mom, years later, I had learned my lesson. I knew what it was like to feel supported by friends, and I wanted to lean on that support. I could survive without it, but I wouldn't be surviving well. I let some friends know what was going on, that I was having a hard time. (When I can't find the words, I have found "I'm having a hard time" conveys what it needs to.) I've learned who steps up can surprise you as much as who doesn't. The friends who knew texted me regularly to check in for updates or just to say they were thinking about me and my mom, and I was grateful to feel less alone.

Though he had spent so much time "suffering in silence" about his mom's care, Ron, as mentioned earlier, has found support from a small circle of friends he holds close. "I have a really, really great best friend who's super supportive over the last couple of years in terms of sharing, like, the day-to-day and just being there. Just to have a caring presence in your life is a game changer and very healing for us."

So how *do* you open up to friends, particularly if you don't think they've experienced something similar themselves? How do you broach it? I took this question to Christina Irving, licensed social worker at Family Caregiver Alliance. Her advice: just start talking about it. Irving said:

> Not everyone will really get it or fully understand your experience right now, but they may end up facing it at some point. It can also help to be clear about what is supportive to you—do you just want them to listen so you can vent or are you wanting some suggestions or ideas from them? It's okay to say, "I just need you to listen and to have your support, but I don't need you to try and come up with solutions." It can also be helpful to let friends know this might impact your ability to stay as connected or to hang out but that you still appreciate hearing from them even if you can't always respond.

MAKING NEW FRIENDS THROUGH SUPPORT GROUPS

As a college student, Feylyn, now a caregiving researcher, heeded the advice to confide in a friend about caring for her mom; she was ready but found her friend wasn't. "I could see she was just like, 'Whoa, this is too much.' And of course now that we're older, now that I'm trained, you realize like the normal—I hate to say 'the normal'—person who is not used to the messiness of disability, care, poverty, the impacts that happen with all of that, they would really be incompetent and unable to hold space for that." If you suspect or find that your peer group is unable to hold space for what you want to share about caregiving, a support group can be a good place to turn. Even if your friends are willing to listen, sometimes you are seeking specific support that your friend group can't fulfill. No matter how present or well-intentioned, if someone isn't in a similar boat or hasn't been, they may not be able to offer the comfort or advice you need. One woman in her thirties didn't know what to anticipate nearing the end of her grandfather's life; she posted to Caregiver Collective asking if someone was emotionally available to help her prepare for hospice. Other members jumped in to share support and experiences, advice they had to impart. Other times, someone just needs to talk to someone else who understands caregiving, so they'll post asking if there's anyone available to chat on the phone. Support group friends may not take the place of your other friendships, but they can fill a desperate hole that needs filling and be a source of reciprocal comfort.

WHAT FRIENDS CAN SAY

If you're the friend on the receiving end, trying to figure out what to say to a person you know in this situation, here's a tip: what caregivers really want is someone—not everyone, just someone—to hear them. Recognize that they are having a hard time, tell them you see them. Empathize and show compassion. It can feel difficult, especially if you haven't experienced anything similar to their situation, so you may be at a loss. That's okay.

"Being authentic can be admitting that you don't know what to say, allowing yourself to be imperfect like that," offered Debbie, who cares for her mom and is also a licensed therapist. "You don't have to be the fixer in the situation. You don't need to have an answer. Because often there's not an easy answer or solutions to some of the stuff caregivers are dealing with. I think it's more about just being present for somebody and really listening. And even if you are just beginning to understand what they're talking about, that's still a really good place to start."

PART THREE

HOW WE'RE FEELING AND WHY IT MATTERS

CHAPTER 10

CAREGIVING AND OUR MENTAL HEALTH

Here are five words any Millennial who grew up in the United States in front of a television will understand: *Jessie Spano, I'm so excited.*

In an old *Saved by the Bell* episode, Jessie, Bayside High's effortless overachiever, is set to perform for music producers with her hot new girl group, Hot Sundae (just go with this). Jessie had a muscly boyfriend who called her "Mama" (Saturday mornings taught us this was a hot commodity in SoCal high schools), her sights set on Stanford, and could lip sync in neon spandex without a hint of embarrassment. Jessie had it all... which, in this episode, also included a caffeine pill addiction. The lesson was that even overachievers, especially overachievers, have a hard time thriving under pressure and expectations; when they do, they can turn to nasty substances. Late for the group's performance and at her breaking point, Jessie, in a famously unhinged outburst, exclaims: "There's no time! There's never any time!" In her bedroom, she breaks into the song she had been expected to perform.

"*I'M SO EXCITED!*" Jessie belts out in the classic meltdown scene, cry-sing-screaming in her best friend Zack's face. "*I'M SO EXCITED! I'm so... scared.*"

Keeping all the plates spinning, terrified of dropping one, at the brink and ready to lose it at a moment's notice: this is the deep inner world of your caregiving peers.

I say *deep inner world* because, most often, this is not what caregivers project or admit even to themselves. To sit with your emotions, really face how you're feeling beyond exhausted, overwhelmed, *There's never any time!*, is to grapple with such profound sadness and fear that, often, we shove right through it. Until we break.

One of my Jessie Spano moments occurred in a wheelchair-accessible minibus cruising across New York's East River. My dad had been talking about wanting to visit Las Vegas, where he lived when he was in high school and where he'd brought me as a teenager to stay at Caesar's Palace whose entire atmosphere suspended reality. I distilled from this Vegas talk that a lot of his desire was to do something splashy and entertaining, to take him out of the day-to-day and transport him to a momentary state of *Whoa!*-inducing amazement. I wasn't sure how I could get him to Nevada, but I did see Cirque du Soleil was in town in New York so bought tickets for the two of us and my mom to go for his birthday. I wasn't making a ton of money at the time but wanted to do something special; I wanted, in essence, to give him joy and awe and to reaffirm my love for him through a special planned event. I arranged wheelchair-accessible seats and scheduled the wheelchair-accessible ride to get us from Manhattan to Queens, where the show was to go on, and made sure it would arrive early to give us plenty of time, just in case. Punctuality was paramount to my father, and he was so strict about it that at times it still comes up for me in therapy.

The van did not arrive early. Or even what I would consider on time-ish. It was late. With each minute we waited by the front door of his nursing home, my skin turned prickly. I was on high alert, my heartbeat in my ears. The kind of stress where you can't properly see or hear, but I was trying to maintain an upbeat, excited demeanor because that's how I wanted the day to go. That's how I had planned the day to go. I had read all the venue's accessibility info in advance, I had filled my purse with the bendy straws my dad needed to safely swallow, we were prepped to smuggle in the thickened cans of Ensure that he could drink and, actually, really enjoyed. (I was most likely not wearing neon spandex, although I can't state this with complete confidence.) I had thought through and done everything I could to make sure this day was smooth and enjoyable, including scheduling early transport, and now the fucking wheelchair-accessible minibus was not here and who knew where it was and...

Then it arrived. Slight relief, until the driver took us completely out of the way. I felt just a complete lack of control. We were on our way, somehow, finally on the move, but who knew when we'd get there or if we'd miss the whole thing. This was my last (bendy) straw. I was frustrated; I was angry. Sitting on the bench seat beside my dad's chair, I burst into tears. My father looked up at me like I was a lunatic. Spectacle and awe, delivered.

We pulled up to the wheelchair-accessible entrance just after the curtain went up. A venue staff member whisked us down a long roped gangway and we flew through back hallways to a door close to the stage. We settled into our cushy accessible seats, a few rows from the stage. The whole thing had a very VIP feeling to it. We cranked our necks up to watch, above us, performers flying and dancing through the air. We bought concession foods from the vendors making their way through the aisles. Throughout the show, my dad asked me if I wanted something else, making sure I had enough to eat. Sitting there with both my parents, hands filled with a hot dog and carton of popcorn, I felt like a kid. I leaned onto the arm of my dad's wheelchair, holding his hand. I felt safe. I was happy.

Irrational outbursts like the one I had on the way to the show became common. So did asking the question "Did I mess up my makeup?" once I calmed down. I didn't want my instability to be seen from the outside via mascara under my eyes or streaked bronzer. I didn't want my instability to be seen. Unpacking my feelings in retrospect, the truth is I was dealing with a lot of heavy emotions and fears, the weight of which felt too much to sit with, to face. This overwhelm rerouted into anger and frustration. Having a Jessie Spano moment followed in the same day by deep unconditional happiness and love also became common. I'd go to bed exhausted from the range of emotions alone.

When I told friends about that day at Cirque du Soleil, I did not share the explosion of tears and instead focused on the good time we had. From the outside, it was a great day with my dad and my mom. And it was. But without sharing the other flood of emotions so present in the day-to-day of caregiving—the anger, sadness, frustration, overwhelm—people in your life are in the dark about your true mental state.

Instead, when people observe the care situation you're in and take a moment to notice how much you are handling, you often hear: *You're so strong.* "You're so strong, I don't know if I could do it." Or "You're so strong, what would they do without you?"

At times, hearing this you feel like a fraud. *They only think I'm strong because they don't see the days I feel broken inside, when I have to splash my face with cold water to depuff my crying eyes before we go to lunch.* Other times, you know they are right. You are strong, despite the rough days. Being told I was strong and being seen that way were affirming, the pep talk I needed. As time went on, though, being strong also felt like a burden I'd been chosen to bear. The strong ones get dealt the tough stuff; the strong ones are expected to shoulder it and keep going. But why couldn't someone else be strong sometimes? Why did it always feel like it had to be me?

What they're actually talking about is resilience.

I think of resilience as the quality of muscling through, like a super-hero who steps into a barrage of bullets, only for each to bounce off their chest with a little *ping!* But for us humans, clinical psychologist George Bonanno defined resilience as "the ability of people who have experienced a highly life-threatening or traumatic event to maintain relatively stable, healthy levels of psychological and physical functioning."[1] It's true: caregivers are resilient. When faced with an unforeseen emergency room visit, an unexpected phone call from an unknown number that makes our stomach churn, the exhaustion of it all, we keep going...even when it feels impossible and like we can't continue.

Millennial resilience, as far as I've seen, has only been studied in the workplace. There, we excel: Millennial leaders were found to have "the ability to bounce back from impediments and hindrances." They also "displayed more maturity and responsibility while handling relationships" than leaders of other generations did.[2] So, as far as performance, Millennials are looking pretty good. Jessie Spano, it should be noted, did get into Stanford. But performance and mental health are clearly two different things. If we apply George Bonanno's definition of resilience to caregiving, are we maintaining, as he put it, psychological and physical functioning through it all? Yes. We take a licking and keep on ticking. But are our levels of functioning healthy?

Understanding the mental health and emotional states of caregivers is important: first, we're human beings undergoing a trying experience. Second, if we're responsible for the mortality of another being, you should be concerned if we're about to have a psychotic break. To really understand the caregivers of our generation, we first need to look at the mental health of Millennials in our country as a whole. Luckily, this topic *has* been given attention by researchers.

The research says we're fucked.

OUR MENTAL HEALTH CRISIS

Millennials have come to be known as the "burnout generation." One study found that, when it comes to mental health, our generation is experiencing a "health shock" (unpredictable illness that diminishes health) on par with the effects AIDS had on the Boomer generation.[3] Although not fully understood, this could be the result of increased isolation and decreased economic security.

Before the pandemic, suicide rates for all Americans were on the rise (including Gen Z).[4] But in the years leading up to the pandemic, the mortality rate of Millennials specifically had increased substantially; we were more likely to die prematurely from suicide or a drug overdose than previous generations were.[5] Stanford University research cites among the reasons "decades-long rising inequality" for our generation (again, the multiple recessions we aged into, the persistent gender gap in equality, systemic racial inequality) and the opioid epidemic. Not only were circumstances low, but expectations for us to succeed were high. Alcohol abuse also rose in the decade leading up to the pandemic: alcohol-related deaths among those ages eighteen to thirty-four were up 69 percent from 2007 to 2017.[6] An article in *The Atlantic* pointed out that people in their twenties and thirties were dying of alcoholic liver disease, which typically takes decades of hard drinking to develop.[7] The caffeine pills were a cautionary tale that couldn't have foreseen the hardships our generation had coming.

Then COVID struck. By late June 2020, 40 percent of American adults were dealing with mental health or substance abuse issues.[8] During this time, it was Millennials and Gen Zers who showed more adverse mental health symptoms than older generations.[9] As one caregiver in her thirties told me, "This whole pandemic experience, it's really worn down on me.... I've been in worse situations with my mom, but for some reason, I was less and less able to cope with the same situation."

A *New York Times* piece on resilience in the face of trauma states, "How we cope depends on what is in our resilience toolbox."[10] Many caregivers our age turned to unhealthy habits as a way to cope: our alcohol and substance use (and abuse) increased during the pandemic.

Now let's add in the stress, fears, and intensified isolation of caregiving. During the pandemic, caregivers' already taxed mental health was put under an entirely new strain and a new norm kicked into gear that required even more intense commitment: most professional home care stopped, people brought office jobs home full-time, physical isolation in order to protect the vulnerable increased, and the only social support was found online. That earlier stat, of how 40 percent of American adults dealt with mental health or substance abuse issues in the first half of 2020? Both unpaid caregivers and younger adults were disproportionately affected.[11]

Caregivers our age who were living with the person they cared for were without a reprieve. Work, care, eating, and sleeping all took place within the same walls. Any personal boundaries that may have existed before the pandemic were eviscerated; access was constant. Getting groceries or going on a walk took on extra fears: if they contracted COVID, it could potentially be brought home to a medically vulnerable person whose health they were already terrified over. Michelle, who was living with her dad and chronically ill mom in a New York City apartment, told me that when lockdown in the city relaxed to stage four, which allowed gatherings of up to fifty people and some indoor dining at restaurants, she remained at, what she called, "stage zero." The risk of communing with others was too high; she was nervous even pushing elevator buttons in her apartment building when she left for a weekly grocery run.

Caregivers who lived apart from the person they cared for also remained vigilant about staying healthy for the day they could visit their loved one. They faced a different set of challenges: with home care effectively stopped, these caregivers had to navigate how their loved one would receive necessary in-home care. For those with loved ones in a facility, they feared the isolation that person had to endure (if the person had dementia, would they think they'd been abandoned?) and the rising mortality rates in nursing homes. The (understandable) fear was so great, many families moved their loved ones out of nursing homes and in with them. Answering one stress by creating another.

The effect on our mental health was staggering. During the pandemic, almost one-third of unpaid family caregivers reported seriously considering suicide.[12] More unpaid family caregivers reported starting or increasing substance use to cope with COVID on top of caregiving.[13] More unpaid family caregivers also reported having depression and anxiety compared to noncaregivers. Among caregivers, these adverse mental health symptoms were twice as high for those who felt unprepared as a caregiver, who did not have the personal freedom they desired, or who had to decrease living expenses to help pay for things, compared to other caregivers.[14]

Our generation's emotional health has not improved since the pandemic. Millennials, Gen Xers, and Gen Zers all report feeling more emotionally distressed.[15] But all of us have shown resilience; we've survived. With the mental health crises our generation (and Gen Z) has faced, and in the wake of the pandemic, the definition of *resilience* may need to be modified. *Functioning at all* seems to be a more reasonable goalpost.

The catch with being called resilient is that it carries with it an implication that we're strong and, because we can stomach it and muscle through, we don't have feelings about what we're witnessing, what we're enduring, what we're missing out on. But instead of projecting and assuming how caregivers feel, how often are they actually asked? And if asked, how often do they respond with honesty?

"Certain friends, family members, like, every single time I see them, one of the first things they'll ask is, 'How's your mom doing?'" Debbie told me. Notice how the question is about how Debbie's *mom* is doing. It's understood that the person who is ailing is the priority, and the question is often born out of care: care for Debbie's mom, and care for Debbie, whose mother is important to her. But what I hear often is that this question replaces asking the caregiver how they themselves are doing. The caregiver is overlooked.

Whereas some take the time to notice our resilience, others don't think about how caregivers feel at all. When Michelle considered donating a kidney to her mother, she noticed that none of the medical professionals in the clinic considered, well, Michelle. She felt their attitude toward the operation was blasé and not a big deal for her to undergo; her well-being wasn't addressed.

"Sometimes I think the experience makes you feel like you don't matter as much. And I think it's really important to continue to put yourself in situations where you do.... This whole experience is what actually made me start seeking out therapy. Because I felt like my needs sort of stopped mattering, like I didn't matter anymore."

ALEXANDRA TOLD ME ABOUT THE "ELABORATE FANTASY" SHE FREQUENTLY had while caring for her mom, who had brain cancer. "What if I just left and I basically went off the grid, but I left my family a note saying, 'I'm fine, but I can't deal with this'? And I would be so ashamed that I would have to change my identity and live in a hut forever.... I would be so guilty. But I thought about that a lot.... It was essentially like I fantasized almost about faking my own death and going back to a simpler version of my life."

A fantasy...about faking her own death. *That* is the honest truth about where the caregiver's head goes. The daydream of running away, returning to a simpler life they had "before," is a common thread I've heard when people do divulge their feelings.

These are the thoughts, the feelings, the emotions that caregivers don't share with friends, with family, or with partners. The people in our life who care about us, who could help, are left in the dark. Instead, we respond to their questions with a too-quick and cheery "I'm good!" or the more grounded "I'm good," and we press on, pushing our feelings down.

Suppressing our feelings around others doesn't mean we're unaware of them. Just the opposite is true: as NPR put it, "Millennials might be the generation of emotional intelligence."[16] We pay attention to how we feel and use that knowledge to self-regulate...or try to. Despite caregivers keeping our feelings to ourselves, our generation is primed to share: Millennials are more likely to talk about mental health than our parents or grandparents were.[17]

Our emotional intelligence is not just for ourselves but also for those we care for. We often take their feelings into account, maybe even taking them on as our own. Michelle and I both cared for parents whose diseases could physically worsen with depression; it puts you on alert for not only noticing how they are feeling but also managing it to prevent their condition from worsening. It's a lot of pressure and an unrealistic responsibility to take on.

HOW CAREGIVERS FEEL, *REALLY*

Multiple people brought up feeling like they were in survival mode. Jesus, who cares for both parents and is particularly learned about caregivers our age, told me how survival mode means our mental health gets pushed to the back burner: "You have all these strains, but you're not at liberty to really be like, 'Hey, this is going on' because you're so caught up in the day-to-day. So those financial and emotional, physical strains, it's like, you just have to deal with it."

In the following chapters, we're going to get honest about the range of emotions I most often hear expressed by caregivers our age. Some (as they relate to caregiving) are particular to our generation; others are not but play out in people our age in unique ways. Emotions such as anxiety, anger, and grief are common responses to trauma, but we're going to discuss their specificity in caregivers our age—where these feelings stem from, what they indicate about our generation as a whole, and healthy ways we can address them.[18]

CHAPTER 11

WE'RE FEELING *ISOLATED AND ALONE*

"IT'S KIND OF SCARY AND LONELY, YOU KNOW, LOOKING AT THE FUTURE so helplessly, not knowing what is going to happen with his health." That's Casey, telling me what it's like navigating her husband's chronic illness, but it could be anyone our age who is caregiving. This feeling of loneliness, of isolation, is a common thread binding pretty much every caregiver I've met.

During the pandemic lockdowns, here's what caregivers our age said behind closed doors, to each other: *Finally, people* get *it.* Not being able to schedule anything social, being confined at home with the person they care for, seeking whatever resources they could online—this isolation was already something caregivers were used to, and now the rest of the world got a taste. Caregivers finally felt a semblance of social equality. Some even said that during lockdowns others became more aware of their situation and, at last, offered some assistance. It got to the point that people in the caregiver group actually lamented a post-lockdown world in which everyone would no longer be in the same boat, the rest of the world back to normal while they remained isolated outliers, once again.

In a paper written on the COVID pandemic and collective trauma, the author cites ongoing isolation as a trauma in itself.[1] There are three main reasons for this: isolation "disrupts patterns of socialization that significantly contribute" to our sense of self; it demands social

distancing that is a "powerful source of anxiety, loneliness and grief";
and it forces us to live with constant fear that we or a loved one will die
alone. All this rings familiar for those who are caregiving, and it has for
a long time. The sense of isolation experienced by caregivers our age is,
it can be deduced, a trauma for young adults in and of itself and needs
to be paid attention. To understand how we can address this among
caregivers, first we need to ask: In this age of collective experiences, why
do we all feel so alone?

A prepandemic study found Millennials to be "the loneliest generation."[2] Almost a third of Millennials surveyed reported that they always
or often feel lonely; more than 20 percent of Millennials said they had
no friends. Studies have pointed to the internet and social media as
main contributors. Although social media seemingly connects people,
research has shown that increased social media use exacerbates feelings of social isolation in young adults.[3] Watching the curated lives of
others, it turns out, can make you feel depressed, and the more images
and stories you take in, the worse you feel. Research also finds that com-
municating digitally, including over FaceTime or WhatsApp, does not
have the same mental health benefits as spending time with others in
person.[4] A study by Harvard found 43 percent of young adults reported
increased loneliness since the outbreak of the pandemic.[5]

Loneliness in our nation has become such a problem that Surgeon
General Vivek Murthy declared it an epidemic in the United States.
Among contributing factors he names the pandemic, a breakdown in
communities and personal connectivity, social media use, and an
increase in judgments and divisions among our population. The effects
on our physical and mental health are profound. "When people are
socially disconnected, their risk of anxiety and depression increases," he
wrote in the *New York Times*. "So does their risk of heart disease (29%),
dementia (50%), and stroke (32%). The increased risk of premature death
associated with social disconnection is comparable to smoking daily—
and may be even greater than the risk associated with obesity."[6] Again, to

put everything into context, Millennials were named the loneliest generation: people our age were already predisposed to feelings of significant loneliness, then found themselves in a further isolating experience of caregiving young.

Caregiving disrupts identity-building social patterns, thrusts us into constant fear over a loved one's health that we don't believe others feel, and restricts us from socially interacting with others, which is lonely. More than half of Millennial caregivers are undergoing the responsibility alone, without anyone to share the experience with.[7]

Michelle, who, you remember, lived at home caring for her mom who had renal failure, told me that when she overheard friends or colleagues her age talking about their lives, their experiences were so different from hers that she didn't dare share what she was going through. We spoke about this earlier in relation to her friendships, but it's part of a larger emotional pattern that leads to turning inward. "I felt like I couldn't relate to my peers," she told me. "When I went to work and everybody was talking about their brunch plans and I'm just like, I was knee-deep with kidney juice. Don't ask me about my weekend.... That's the other thing, too, because then it's like, do you want to be the Debbie Downer in the group? But that's your reality. And so you just sort of get comfortable with saying, like, 'Oh, it's fine. My weekend was fine.'"

Her social isolation increased when plans with friends got put on the back burner and eventually fizzled out. She prioritized being with her mom and taking care of her mom's needs; when she did have time available, she was so exhausted from care work and her career that she just wanted to sleep. That physical distance from her friends compounded her emotional distance, from them and people her age in general. "You become less able to relate socially, you get a little bit more isolated, and then it reinforces this isolation of caregiving too, right? I remember early on in the pandemic we started talking about the isolation that people were feeling from not going out, not being social. I was like, I'm kind of used to this. This is sort of like our reality."

SOCIAL MEDIA: HELP OR HURT?

Then there's social media, reinforcing the lives we're not living with images and cute music-driven videos. Caregivers absorb social media differently, believing their own experience is one really no one relates to, while friends are living seemingly carefree lives. "Seeing my friends go to festivals I had tickets to or out for fun date nights or these kinds of things...it just made me jealous," Alexandra said when I asked about her social media use. I wanted to talk to Alex particularly because, as a travel blogger and influencer, social media plays a large part in her work life. Despite being online, she said that while she was caregiving for her mom with brain cancer, she "backed away" from her friends' social media posts. "I didn't want to resent them for just living their wonderful lives.... On a one-on-one basis, I didn't feel that way. I had friends get engaged and have all these exciting things happen in their life while I was taking care of my mom. Maybe because it was the more human-to-human personal connection, I wasn't resentful of them at all. But somehow scrolling through on a screen and seeing everyone you've ever met in your life having a good time just made me...while I'm sitting on the couch watching *Law and Order*, something which I used to love to do, but when you have no other option for so long, it's a little less so."

One thing about my conversation with Alex I found so interesting is that while social media made her feel disconnected from friends in a way that connecting with them in person did not, it was also a platform she used to open up about her feelings of caregiving for her mom. At the time, she was one of the few caregivers our age I observed being publicly candid about what she was going through; I asked her why she decided to first post about it. "I felt very isolated," she told me. "As much as we were surrounded by my mom's incredible community that she really spent her entire life cultivating...I was going through all these crazy moments of self-discovery, anticipatory grief, and loneliness. Writing has always been how I connected with the world, and my mom was a writer, so it's how she connected with the world too. So I think just starting to vulnerably share some of that...it kind of made me feel a little sane again." On the one hand, social media had enflamed some "negative" emotions observing the lives of friends, but on the other hand, Alex used it as a tool to express her own experience. Feelings of isolation up, feelings of isolation down, depending on its use.

What was the response to such heavy material? "Really overwhelmingly supportive," Alex said. There was no downside to her career, although some family members did not approve of her public share. She received a lot of messages from people around her own age living a similar experience, and she was "shocked" to find how many of us there are. I asked if this online connection through her story helped to combat her own feelings of isolation.

"It did in some ways, yeah," Alex said. "It was hard reading some people's journeys, but I think it did help in some way. It kind of gave me some sense of purpose, especially when I was getting so many messages from people telling me how much it meant to them to hear from someone else going through the same thing....Someone being like, 'I'm going through this crazy hard time' made them feel less alone." From Alex's response, it sounds like being honest and vulnerable online did have some positive effect on alleviating her personal sense of isolation, but the larger emotional response was experienced by others who absorbed her story in their feed. It demonstrates, I believe, a desire of people living through a hard time (particularly one they feel others don't relate to) to see that experience reflected by others online.

LONGING FOR CONNECTION

This longing to see themselves mirrored in another person and to have someone to relate to is something I found to be at the root of the isolation and disconnect I heard caregivers express.

"I had been dealing with a significant lack of connection and isolation for years by dealing with this experience alone," Ron said. Remember, Ron had been caring for his mother in one way or another since he was a teenager. Once he became an adult and began his career, the disconnect with others his age only became more apparent when he encountered how they would spend their time after work. "When folks are going out for happy hour or when folks were, you know, talking about what I used to deem 'frivolous' things. Now I realize they were just age-appropriate things.... You really end up not really relating to folks who are like, 'Oh, work is done. What should I go do, like, should I go hang out?'...I was not living that life at all. I was living a completely different life." Instead of building personal relationships with people at work, he kept most details about his home life to himself. He felt that people weren't that interested in hearing about his role at home. He said the "human instinct to connect" with others was something he craved after so many years of keeping to himself, feeling isolated and alone. "I think at some point that clicked and I realized that's what I want, is to be seen by someone in this world for what I deal with and what I go through. So it allowed me to share and then, twofold, as I started to mature, other people were starting to fall into some version of caregiving." He said that as people responded that they were also dealing with something similar, the response made him want to share more. He became a person someone else related to, and it was mutually helpful.

Still, the feelings of disconnection can persist, particularly when caregivers funnel their life experience and ability to relate not only by their caregiving early in life, but also by other factors like gender or marriage status. Ron felt the stratification of his upbringing.

"Sometimes people had both parents," Ron said of the people who reciprocated with their own stories. "Sometimes people's parent got sick, but they had tons of money so that helped them. And I always still felt a little bit on edge where, you know, my dad died. I had to take care of my mom [including] financially....I would start to isolate even further."

SUPPORT GROUP: YAY OR NAY

It can be incredibly validating to feel acknowledged by others who understand the experience you're having. Enter: the support group. One major reason I created Caregiver Collective was because I recognized the lapse in support dedicated to people our age: how we communicate, how caregiving shapes our experience and maturation, how we navigate medical systems, and where we instinctively look for assistance. Christina Irving, the social worker I mentioned, said support groups are a good place to find those people who can mirror your experience back to you, which allows you to view your care work through a light of accomplishments rather than negatives or the to-do list swirling in your brain. (On a practical note: Although they are not for everyone, support groups can also be a great place to find crowdsourced information on particular conditions, which can be immensely helpful, particularly for illnesses in which there is less medical information and insight available.)

Michelle attended a support group of working women who were also caregivers. Though she felt a disconnect because they were older (in their fifties) and in a different stage of their lives, she also found they offered what she didn't know she needed: "They were really supportive and they were telling me how great of a daughter I was. And I was like, Okay, thank you. I needed that. I just needed to hear that."

Brandon told me about the Parkinson's support group he joined, which was filled with "lovely" women in their sixties that he called his Golden Girls. "They were so wonderful. I'm still friends with some of them in it. I learned so much through that. From them, I really did get a pretty good picture of what to expect [of disease progression] and what to try to set up." Still, like Michelle, he felt that disconnect of being the only younger adult caring for a parent; he found Caregiver Collective online because he was hoping to connect with other caregivers his own age. Now he "knows" many, and he's pretty active in our group and the caregiving community in general; still, he's spoken to me about how he doesn't know guys his own age who are caregiving. It's another boundary to true connection he's up against.

Ron also felt disconnected when attending caregiver support groups, even when attendees were close to his age; in his experience, these groups were either predominantly female or dedicated to working women. Gender, he says, is a big reason he continues to feel disconnected from other caregivers. "I don't feel reluctant to share, but I do think I still feel that aloneness. That nobody really understands, right?" he said. "Because there's a community forming, and it's not big, but it exists, of (I feel) women who are in this situation.... It's very rare to find single, youthful men caregiving." When it comes to younger unmarried guys who are caregiving, Ron said, "I don't think I've met one."

This struck me because Ron and Brandon know each other. They are both single guys of the same generation, who both have lived in New York and care for their moms, and through Caregiver Collective, they've both attended the same online Support Chats. I reminded Ron about Brandon and there was some recognition; he said he resonates with Brandon's posts. These are not forgetful guys, they aren't self-punishing, and they both actively seek connection. So, what is it about the experience of caregiving that, even when we do find people we can relate to and with whom we might find a sense of comfort, we still feel like the emotional heft is ours alone? Or that we don't belong in the group we found? Why do feelings of alienation persist?

"Some of it comes to what that typical picture is and how caregiving is often presented when you look at media," Christina Irving said. "If somebody doesn't see themselves in that picture of caregiving...it might create that mental block of 'that's not who a caregiver is, so I don't know any male caregivers.'... [Relatable representations are] not what comes to their mind, so it might be harder to even think about who else is doing it."

From the viewpoint of someone who has experienced caregiving and who runs a support group with over a thousand caregiving members, I have some advice: When looking for a support network, don't worry so much that you (or they) don't fall into very specific boxes; it's more important to look for the common threads. If you're a caregiver who is also a parent and believes a single-parent support group would provide tips on how to manage work with care or with children, join. Take away the information that could help. You may not find a one-stop shop of community (or maybe you do!), but the few sources of connection you can cobble together might complete a puzzle that you relate to. And, if you're emotionally able, be vocal about your reality. In Caregiver Collective, when people connect with others with honesty about what they are going through, I can practically feel their emotional weight lifted. If people our age are vocal about caregiving, more people will know what is happening in our own society. In the big picture of our dialogue, lack of awareness and support for Millennial caregivers deepens the chasm of our lonely situation; it's why we should confront the reasons we hold back this information about ourselves and if that is actually serving us.

PHYSICAL ISOLATION AND REBUILDING CONNECTION

Aside from the undeniable alienation caregivers our age often feel, we also need to address the physical isolation. The pandemic was such a severe period of physical isolation that, even now, years later, some caregivers are still shadowed by it.

Casey, who cares for her immunocompromised husband, remains physically isolated from others because of his condition. He "is just so severely immunocompromised, and none of the rest of my family is worried about germs at all, and they're just constantly sick. I don't think I've seen my sisters since they got married." The situation leaves Casey without much in-person contact; she works remotely and is, as she put it, "essentially housebound" with him. Once they were engaged, she couldn't tell the people important to her in person so instead shared the news over Zoom. But even these virtual announcements took months to accomplish with his illness; while people resumed their lives she felt "left behind" with news she was so excited about. Not being able to Zoom friends and family to tell them about the engagement because of his low energy, she told me at the time, "feels very isolating."

The physical isolation that can result from caregiving—either in drastic circumstances like Casey's or in less extreme cases, like when a caregiver just can't find the time to see their friends or socialize at all in light of care responsibilities—is something we cannot sweep under the rug as a dismissible casualty of caregiving. Limited face-to-face contact nearly doubles someone's risk of having depression.[8] In-person connection is necessary for the caregiver's health.

However, when physical connection is limited or impossible, Casey recommends online support groups; she said they've really helped her. Casey is incredibly thoughtful so, in speaking with me, pointed out how supportive Caregiver Collective has been to her. "Joining support groups, I think, is so important. I think we live in a wonderful time where so much is accessible remotely, right? If we were caregiving ten, fifteen years ago—and bless the people who have gone through that—but you're just so isolated, right? And so you can [now access] support, where you can talk to people online.... I think everyone's caregiving situation is just so unique, but there are so many things that we can all still share together."

In our Zoom conversations, Casey used the opportunity to ask me questions about my caregiving history. I think she was genuinely curious and caring, but she also wanted to know how I had dealt with issues similar to hers, like the shifting identity of the person you care for. Our interviews became a bit of a support group meeting in themselves—and Casey wasn't the only one. I noticed other caregivers were both curious and motivated to chat with me as someone with a shared experience; their desire for personal, relatable connection in those moments caught me, admittedly, by surprise but was a source of mutual connection I appreciated right back.

"WE HAVE TO TAKE STEPS IN OUR PERSONAL LIVES TO REBUILD OUR CONnection to one another—and small steps can make a big difference," Surgeon General Murthy advises in that *New York Times* piece. "This is medicine hiding in plain sight:... It could be spending 15 minutes each day to reach out to people we care about, introducing ourselves to our neighbors, checking on co-workers who may be having a hard time, sitting down with people with different views to get to know and understand them, and seeking opportunities to serve others, recognizing that helping people is one of the powerful antidotes to loneliness."[9]

From a Millennial caregiver's perspective, I know how each of us can get wrapped up in our own lives: caregivers can be consumed with keeping the wheels from falling off the metaphorical hospital gurney while replying to a boss's emails or looking for a new job. The noncaregivers in our lives can be consumed with whatever version of that preoccupation exists in their own lives. But I've learned connecting is a mutual responsibility, and that lesson has only been validated through these conversations I've had with caregivers. While writing this book, I had an intense period of simultaneous family medical crises. It was a chronically terrifying time. Once again, I felt totally alone as the only child of a parent whose health had sent up a massive red flare. But this time I took a lesson from caregiving for my dad: I reached out to friends. I was honest about what was happening and how upset I was—it didn't require many words. If I couldn't speak it out loud because I thought it would make me feel more upset, I texted the information. Once friends knew what I was going through, they checked up on me.

Caregivers: Keep the people in your life filled in on your situation. To the people who care about someone whose family member is in questionable health or ability: Check in with them regularly. A simple formula that can make a world of difference toward all of us feeling more connected to each other:

Fill in.
Check in.
Fill in.
Check in.
Fill in.
Check in.

CHAPTER 12

WE'RE FEELING *STRESSED*

After about a year, I was just—I admitted I was not okay....I'd never had a panic attack before and then I had several back to back and I had no idea what was going on. One of my friends told me what a panic attack felt like, so at least I knew it wasn't a heart attack, because it felt like [that].

—Casey, 35

ASEY'S PANIC ATTACKS BEGAN WHEN IT WAS THOUGHT HER FIANCÉ had end-stage liver disease. This is just one example of how stress manifests for us. Caregiving and stress are practically synonymous, but unless you've experienced caregiving yourself, you may not understand how deep that stress runs. Pre-COVID, 80 percent of caregivers ages eighteen to thirty-nine reported that providing care translated to stress levels from moderate to severe—this is higher than our Gen X or Boomer counterparts.[1] We need to ask ourselves: Why are Millennials experiencing this stress so acutely?

Let's first look at our culture as a whole. Burnout, the result of excessive and prolonged emotional, mental, and physical stress, is on the rise.[2] The groups found to be most stressed? Millennials, Gen Z, and women.[3] So that's our baseline. We're balancing work and family and the fallout of multiple financial crises...all the stressors for our generation I've already mentioned are in play. On top of that, Millennials have high expectations for ourselves—we strive for perfection at higher levels than previous generations do.[4] That's a lot of pressure to shoulder when the blocks have already been stacked like a late-stage game of Jenga. Even more pressure when you apply this perfectionism to caring for a chronically ill or ailing person, which we do.

And let's add on the stress of seeing someone you love grapple with failing health. When Millennial caregivers were asked about the causes of their stress, the health of the person they care for was top of list.[5] Uncertainty about the trajectory of the illness throws our brain into a constant minefield of questions: *Will it get better? Much worse? How soon?* Without predicting the future, you can't rely on an answer, only hope. Even getting a correct diagnosis can be a long journey. When my dad first went to a neurologist after displaying some weird neurological signs, and then falls became regular instead of random, he was diagnosed with Parkinson's. I was, strange to say, relieved. People, a lot of people, had gone through Parkinson's before and, according to TV and magazines, Parkinson's seemed like a disease you live well with. Actor Michael J. Fox has had Parkinson's for decades and he was still working, still *alive*. My dad was in good shape, still independent with only a few noticeable changes, so we caught it early. This Parkinson's diagnosis, in my mind, meant life would be different but it was a disease we could manage. There was a known regimen to be followed. My dad started on meds, and we checked in on how they were working. At first they seemed to help; again, tentative relief. Maybe this was what pharmaceuticals do! Stop disease in its tracks, reverse it so someone is back to their old self. I'd never been in a situation like this before, but so far it was looking like a best-case scenario. After a few months, though, we stopped seeing any improvement.

Oh fuck, now what?

Back to the neurologist, this time *the* specialist, *the* expert at *the* hospital. He believed my dad had PSP. Like Parkinson's, but worse. Seemingly rare, usually fatal. A disease with a ticking clock (my thought: *Not on my watch*). Not much was known about the disease, in fact, so little that it's often misdiagnosed first as Parkinson's or never diagnosed at all. New meds, physical therapy, and exercise were critical. So was maintaining my dad's mood: with PSP, depression could actually degrade his physical condition in a way he might not come back from. Keeping up with medications, keeping him moving in meaningful ways, keeping him happy—this was the to-do list I took on. I didn't think twice. I felt the stress tighten my insides, but I don't think I mentally registered it. Not at first.

You can work and pray for your dad's or sister's or husband's health to improve, hope that the illness turns around enough to be easily manageable and less painful, pray that they get better completely; or, at a certain point, you just fight to keep it from getting any worse. At least when there's stasis in the new normal, you can manage a semblance of control. Abrupt or unexpected declines in a person's condition feel like the ground is falling out from under you. Empathy for the seriously ill is biologically hardwired into our brains; according to the National Institutes of Health (NIH), a neurological mechanism within us tells us to do what we can to end someone else's suffering.[6] Caregivers are always grappling with that primal motivation to do anything to help our loved one, to save them. What we don't tell you is we think it's our responsibility and we think we can, despite when logic dictates otherwise. Feeling comfortable is dangerous because at any moment something may happen—a fall, a new symptom—and you'll need to snap into action.

That uncertainty triggers anxiety of always waiting for the other shoe to drop. It's a form of heightened vigilance, a shield that's hard to put down.

"It makes you hyperaware of your surroundings and the people in your community who are in these situations," Jesus said. Does that elderly person on the stairs need help? Is someone with a cane struggling to open a door? My eyes and mind spring into action the moment I sense something, while my conversation with you might continue. When you're used to things popping up, you can't relax; there's a constant threat of danger. Fight-or-flight mode is activated at all times. To alleviate our own stress, even subconsciously, we try to place controls on things.

Brandon described the year of "endless tests and experimental treatments and exploratory surgery" to figure out why his mom was experiencing debilitating pain. With her eventual Parkinson's diagnosis, he tried to get a handle on organization and control in managing her care. (I just want to note: I've since learned Parkinson's is not as rosy a disease as *People* magazine had me thinking it was.)

> *I had a little checklist, you know. I thought we would just set up the new normal.... We thought we'd be able to figure out some breezy new thing.... I mean, I think like so many of these things, though: you fix one problem and another one pops up and then while you're doing that, you discover these three other problems that are there.*

Stress from uncertainty and fear of the unknown is also transposed onto our own lives when we don't know what the future looks like for ourselves. The time and attention care requires can make job futures feel uncertain, and for caregivers that is *stressful*. If they lost their job, what about health insurance? What about income? Employment and financial challenges were found to be consistent sources of stress for Millennial caregivers, as was not feeling like we are getting needed support from our workplace, school, family, friends, or healthcare team.[7]

When Casey was experiencing panic attacks, she was working full-time at the graphic design job she had held since before the pandemic and before her husband's illness. When everyone else returned to the office, she remained working remotely to protect his health. It was her way of balancing his care with continuing her career. At first, she felt grateful that her boss allowed her to work from home but then noticed discrepancies between herself and everyone else in the company. They were offered raises and extra benefits that she wasn't; in-office colleagues celebrated each other's birthdays while hers went overlooked. She felt like the "odd stepchild that nobody thinks about until they need something."

It both put Casey on edge and made her feel inferior, like she was lucky to keep her job at all—despite having been there for nine years and being more experienced than newer hires. She lost sleep working extra hours to make up for the missed work hours spent at doctor appointments and had no time to decompress. She said counseling taught her how to deal with the panic attacks as they were happening, with breathing techniques and retraining her brain not to spiral. They helped, but did not alleviate her psychological state entirely.

Casey was diagnosed with adjustment disorder with depression. Adjustment disorder is a stress-related condition in which there's an excessive reaction to a stressful or traumatic event that involves negative thoughts, strong emotions, and changes in behavior (like panic attacks).[8] Millennial caregivers are more likely to experience stress-related conditions than other generations are. Adjustment disorder and hypertension are 82 percent more prevalent for us than for the "typical" American.[9]

When I spoke with Casey a year later, she had found a different job with a new boss who, to her incredible surprise, helped her to feel supported both as an employee and as a caregiver by encouraging Casey to take occasional paid days off for her own rest:

> *Just yesterday my manager instant-messaged me and she was like, "Hey, hear me. I know you've been dealing with a lot of stress, but why don't you just take a day or two off just to rest, just for you. Not for tasks, not for caregiving, not for running in to the doctor." And I was like, Are you an angel?*

I asked Casey how her stress and anxiety are now.

"I haven't had a single panic attack since I left my old job."

BALANCING IT ALL

Caregiving Millennials were asked to name what stressed them specifically, and their answers were an overlap of caregiving and noncaregiving stress contributors.[10] In other words, they were stressed by balancing caregiving with other aspects of their lives, such as career or kids or their own needs. Ask a caregiver when they last saw a doctor for their own well-being.

During the pandemic, Michelle, who lived with her parents to care for her mom, continued working her full-time job remotely. While the world struggled to comprehend the gravity of the pandemic, Michelle was doing that and caregiving without the personal space her work office had provided. With that boundary gone, Michelle's parents had unlimited access to her without barriers. They would pop into her room with questions while she was on a company Zoom meeting. They asked her daily to run errands, such as to the post office, that she didn't see as essential. Walking out of her bedroom meant facing regular requests from her parents. She found herself working online well past the time when everyone else was signing off and often stayed working until she fell asleep—she was using work to escape the home life just a room away. Michelle's interim solution: she hung a "Do Not Disturb" sign on her door.

She sought therapy; a few virtual game nights with friends helped, until they tapered off as people settled into quarantine fatigue. But even when the pandemic waned, the compounded effects of her stress were still present and in fact were building. She hit a breaking point, her second instance of caregiver burnout.

"I think it's the buildup of the pandemic and just unhealthy coping mechanisms. . . . I was like, I need to get out. I need to change my environment. And I need to do it safely." She had already considered the idea of renting her own apartment just before lockdown started and, in its wake, realized her need for her own space was dire. One year into the pandemic is when she booked that three-month Airbnb just a few blocks from her parents' home. Temporarily moving into the private space didn't eliminate her stress—far from it—but did allow her a reprieve and a quiet place of her own to come down. Her own needs may not have been fully in balance with everything else, but they were back in the equation.

UNCERTAINTY

Uncertainty about competency and abilities as a caregiver is also high on the Millennial caregiver stressor list.[11] Young caregiving adults might not have ever been fully responsible for another human before—let alone someone ailing with specific, and evolving, care needs. There's a steep learning curve for anyone, and feeling inexperienced adds to the stress. If you don't have someone your own age to model the experience for you, to give practical advice or emotional support, this sense of being in over your head makes an already stressful job even more so. When my dad's throat muscles weakened and swallowing became an issue, it wasn't just a matter of helping him to eat; I was doing it with the stress of knowing that if something was not cut up small enough, or was too small, it could go down the wrong pipe and into his lungs and cause pneumonia and he could die. It was a cause of death we were warned about. That is freaking stressful, and that's just daily eating.

Not to mention some of the practical medical demands expected of caregivers: Michelle disinfected her hands and everything in the apartment daily to help run her mom's dialysis machine; Lea had to learn how to change her mom's colostomy bags at home. There are many, many ways in which we're feeling in over our heads and praying it all goes right.

DISRUPTION

Disruptions to your life outside of your control and needing to make sudden adjustments are unwelcome realities of caregiving; so is the impact it may have on younger caregivers hitting life milestones. The uncertainty caused by significant disruptions to our achievements and functioning was found to be another cause of stress among caregivers in our generation. This happens with the big things, such as: *Will I be able to meet a partner and actually maintain a relationship while caregiving is my foreseeable future? Do I have to drop out of grad school because my professors don't recognize caregiving as an excuse for missing class and now I'm behind in credits?* But it can also feel like a constant state of being, waiting for something else to happen that will interrupt the plans we've managed to make; to counteract this, to stanch the bleeding, we try to put safety control measures into place.

When Brandon and his brother, both living in New York, realized their mom could no longer live alone in her Michigan house, "We just kept coming up with plans and we didn't know all the information," he said. "So we'd have these plans and they wouldn't...just all the facts would change and then you're making another plan, and quickly." In hindsight, knowing what he knows now, some of the plans they cooked up in the moment were "completely insane"; in truth, they were doing the best they could in evolving circumstances.

Caregivers are always paranoid about the other shoe dropping because, often, we're hearing a shoe hit the floor in the other room. A shoelace breaks and you're busy researching Velcro when you get a phone call that the shoe has burst into flames. Before Debbie's mom moved into assisted living, Debbie felt on edge with her mom living at home alone:

I had a lot of anxiety...kind of like developing that response of just, like, always waiting for the other shoe to drop, basically. Like always feeling like you have to be on alert. Or, you know, looking at my phone and seeing a bunch of missed calls from my mom and thinking, Is this a crisis? And just kind of not knowing, it was a roller coaster. It's still a roller coaster.

The phone ringing was a huge anxiety trigger for me, too; in my case, with unknown numbers. Was it a hospital? A nursing home administrator? Every spam call made my skin hurt, my nerves erupting while I tried to remain calm. At times, I'd actually feel breathless listening to a message from an unknown caller. The knowledge that something awful you didn't foresee happening (or worse, that you did) could actually happen is a constantly simmering stress the entire time you are caregiving; in my experience, it lasts long after, too. Even though I'm not caregiving, these phone calls still prick my attention and I have slight fear something bad has happened to someone I love.

RELATIONSHIP DYNAMICS

Millennial caregivers also cited relationship dynamics, both with the person they care for and others in their lives, as a cause of their stress.

Some caregivers already have a tense relationship with the person they care for before providing care begins. Several caregivers in my group are caring for alcoholic parents they've had a tumultuous relationship with for most of their lives; it doesn't stop them from providing care now that the parent is ill, but it also hasn't improved their relationship or eased resentment. Others find the relationship strained because of the illness: print ads and commercials I see in New York about becoming a paid family caregiver show, usually, a grandmother and daughter or granddaughter embracing each other, talking about how great it is to spend all day together. They don't depict Grandma throwing something across the room or being verbally abusive in a dementia episode or forgetting to turn off the stove—all instances that can regularly happen with disease and can create an emotional block between the family members or instigate the caregiver's own stress spiral.

"I think that's part of dementia, just how rapidly someone's mood can change and how disoriented and distressed someone can become," Debbie told me about her mom's unpredictable moods. "Trying to stay level myself and kind of not get on the roller coaster with her has been an ongoing challenge for me that I've had to really, really work on so that at least one of us is staying not too stressed out in this situation."

HEALTHCARE SYSTEM

One major source of the mental load so many caregivers I spoke with had in common was dealing with the healthcare system. It's exhausting: phone call after phone call to insurance companies, trying to figure out which exact treatments are covered and how many, whether you can get an extension in coverage when physical therapy sessions run out but your person needs more. It can feel like there is always a call to make and answers given that you just cannot wrap your brain around.

"Changing somebody, the hygiene care for somebody, making sure they're okay...that's tough. But the paperwork stuff, always, is brutal." This was Jesus, talking about caring for his mom. "Phone calls that you know the kind of no's that you'll get, knowing that you have a loved one who's in dire need of this help and they're telling you 'no' or 'go somewhere else' or 'go call another number.'" When your family's health depends on getting the services that require these calls, it can be the last straw. And. It's. All. The. Time. It's the piece that you assume will be the most manageable, have sense and a system behind it. It's bureaucracy, not heartache, right? Instead, it's another instance in which we don't have control. For Jesus, it's that his sense of urgency is not being reciprocated by someone else.

Remembering my own similar instances, I noticed Jesus and I had a different stress response to bureaucratic medical scenarios. Jesus has empathy for the workers on the other end because, he thinks, they're stressed too and going through their own thing. I had zero patience for anybody when I was in those situations; my stress completely stole the show. While he had awareness to stay tempered despite it being stressful for him, I had a primal fear kick in that, if something in my home system got disrupted, there was going to be a major disruption with my dad's health. I confided to Jesus that, at the time, I was really losing it on people regularly.

"Those things are bound to happen," he told me. "You almost have to give yourself some credit and be like, 'Hey, this happened. It's not ideal.'" Give myself some grace and an opportunity to handle it better next time. Even so many years later, his support was comforting.

CAREGIVER BURNOUT

Caregiver burnout is defined as a state of deep physical, emotional, and mental exhaustion that happens while you're taking care of someone else.[12] Here are symptoms, according to the Cleveland Clinic and displayed by a lot of the people I've spoken with. If you're experiencing some or all these symptoms, you can take this as your red flag to seek help:

- Emotional and physical exhaustion
- Withdrawal from friends and loved ones
- Loss of interest in activities you previously enjoyed

- Feeling hopeless and helpless
- Changes in appetite or weight
- Changes in sleep patterns
- Inability to concentrate
- Getting sick more often
- Irritability/frustration/anger toward others

One of the contributors to burnout is not realizing that burnout is happening. The exhaustion can be confusing when you are sleeping enough hours but still wake up feeling tired and have a hard time shaking it through the day. You can go through periods when it feels unending. This can be emotional exhaustion, which is also common and understandable when dealing with something like chronic illness and a loved one's health. If you are feeling deeply tired, pay attention: you may be experiencing burnout, and it's best to get ahold of it as soon as you can.

What are some other causes of burnout? When caregiving leads us to neglect ourselves... When we bounce between the experience being rewarding or bonding while simultaneously stressful (termed "the varied expectations of caregiving")... When, as discussed earlier, there's role confusion and you have difficulty separating your role as a caregiver from that of being a daughter/son/spouse/friend. It seems to me that these blurred lines can lead us to overextend and lose sight of ourselves. (There can also be increased stress when multiple people are providing care and the roles are unclear; blurred lines and too many cooks in the kitchen cause stress for everyone.)... When there are too many responsibilities... When you feel a lack of control because you don't have the finances, resources, or skills needed to effectively plan, manage, and organize care as you'd want. I hear this a lot when a caregiver knows a home health aide would really help lighten their load or there's a great nursing home they'd trust with their family member's life, but high costs prohibit them from getting the help they know is available to others. It's not just stress but also feeling like there's nothing you yourself can do about it— the helplessness—that stretches you thin.

Another burnout contributor: working in a service-related field, such as in a school or hospital. Kaci, who is a teacher, told me she experienced caregiver burnout. I asked what she thought led to her reaching that point:

Managing, because I do most everything; I do the paperwork, I do the med-ications, I do, like, the actual physical care. I have my mom living with me, I have to do her shopping, I have to manage her money. I have to do all that and I think sometimes it gets to the point that it's just too much and I have to, like, sleep for two days.

Both of the roles she balances, work and home, are in service to others and necessitate strategic planning. Unlike caregiving, her job as a teacher actually grants her some time off. When she's at work, her mother attends a day program that provides care, but in the weeks she has off from work, her mom knows that Kaci is home, so she wants to be home, too. Kaci has worked to convince herself that it's okay for her mom to still attend the day program when Kaci is off work so that Kaci can have those afternoons for herself.

You're also more at risk for burnout if you think no one can provide the care or do the specific task but you and/or you don't have a support system to relieve you when you're tired. How often have I heard, or felt, *It's just easier to do it myself.* Sometimes with medical care it can feel too daunting to fill someone else in on your routine so they can cover for you. Kaci told me that when her brother steps in to help with their mom, it requires her to do so much planning (charts outlining medications, dos-ages, schedules) that she'd rather not pass off the task; doing it herself takes less time. But it's this thought pattern that puts a caregiver at risk of doing too much and doing it all the time.

Once you recognize it, there are ways to alleviate caregiver burnout. It doesn't have to live with you for as long as your role of caregiver does. You are not a better or more devoted person because caregiving has worn you thin and you've given it every ounce of your soul. The opposite.

"In an ideal world, we find ways to prevent it [burnout] from happen-ing," Christina Irving said. It's helpful to get support for burnout early on, she advised, but also recognized that a caregiver might not realize they're in the depths of burnout until they see that list of symptoms. Ask yourself: What can I do for myself right now? "Getting breaks is helpful," Irving said. "How accessible that is really varies based on what public benefits they're eligible for, what community resources exist, where they live, whether they have family or friends that can step in and provide that help.... Exploring that is important." Taking these breaks or accepting outside help hinges on two factors: setting boundaries with the person you care for by expressing to them your need for help, and getting over your own mental obstacles of letting someone step in for you. Remember that letting someone help you, well, helps you.

Respite programs that allow you to get away for a day can help, but they're not the only solution. "A lot of it is building up people's resilience and their capacity to cope with it, which often is these very small things [to care for themselves] that maybe don't feel like they're impactful in the moment," Irving said. "But over time, the cumulative effect does make a difference and they're things that are more realistic for caregivers.... How do you find those little things that you can do that bring you a sense of wellness or joy or peace or relaxation, even if they are brief? Because when you do them often enough, it does make a difference." She suggests finding even five minutes at the start or end of your day for journaling, meditation, or prayer. Incorporate a few more minutes throughout your day to help you destress: put on music while you wash dishes, get outside in nature, play with your pet, spend a few minutes calling a friend. Casey mentioned that her therapist taught her breathing exercises that have helped. When your burnout reaches a dangerous point, counseling is the critical next step of treatment.

It's not just burnout; caregiver stress shows up in other ways.

Compassion Fatigue

According to the Cleveland Clinic, compassion fatigue occurs when the caregiver takes on the emotional stress and trauma of the person they're caring for.[13] Although it sounds like extreme empathy, it can actually lead to a loss of empathy or lack of care for the other person. The NIH expands a bit on compassion fatigue, saying caregivers feeling the pain and suffering of the patient lose a sense of themselves and their role in care.[14] I notice this when I ask a caregiver how they're doing, and they respond by answering how *the person they care for* is doing. Or when I ask a caregiver about their experience and they tell me a bit about their experience but then override the conversation with how badly they feel because the person they care for is depressed or sad or fatigued, and they spend much more time and detail focused on the other person's feelings. They neglect their own emotions and lose sight of themselves out of empathy preoccupation for the other person.

Decision Fatigue

According to the American Medical Association (AMA), decision fatigue is "a state of mental overload that can impede a person's ability to continue making decisions."[15] According to NIH, the typical American makes thirty-five thousand decisions per day.[16] The more decisions you need to make, the harder it is to make further decisions. It gets exhausting. Now apply that to keeping your grandparent alive with your healthcare decision-making. Every option must be weighed for every scenario and the outcomes are particularly high stakes. Even the low-stakes decisions feel major when it's in the context of someone else's well-being.

While writing this book, my uncle's health took a massive downturn because of his Parkinson's and within weeks he passed away. During that intense period of driving down to Virginia with my mom to be with him and my aunt, there were constant decisions to navigate, and quickly: *We know what the doctors say, but do the ways he looks and sounds match that? What are we seeing? Should we try to encourage him to eat? Is he too cold sitting outside, or are the fresh air and bird sounds more important? How long should we stay? Is it safe for us to drive back to New York, or will he deteriorate even more?* My mom and aunt were his primary caregivers, but the exhaustion of it all, particularly when combined with long bedside hours, was a lot for me, too. I remember sitting in front of a diner menu thinking, I'll just eat *whatever.* Did the random order include something I'm allergic to? Please just bring it. I'd rather eat around it than decide what to ask for. Decisions about myself were the most easily discarded.

Signs of decision fatigue include difficulty with focusing and clarity of thought (personally, I experience this as brain fog or extreme distraction), procrastinating often and then making decisions impulsively, avoiding or overthinking decisions, being irritable or having a quick temper, and feeling overwhelmed or hopeless. There are also some physical signs, like poor sleep, fatigue (notice a trend in our stress?), headaches, and other physical ailments.[17]

An article on Care.com helpfully lists the factors that can put you at risk for decision fatigue.[18] According to Barbara Rube, a board-certified expert in traumatic stress, these factors include overload of how many decisions need to be made, decisions that cause grief due to the potential outcome of those choices (caregivers really feel this one, especially when in the role of medical proxy—on the far end of the spectrum is a decision as grave as "Should I keep this person on life support?"), feeling burdened by being the only person capable of making that difficult decision on the other's behalf, and making a decision that goes against your values and moral beliefs but having no choice but to do it.

I've noticed a lot of caregivers turn to my group for help crowdsourcing solutions. Although they won't make the decision for you, support groups can be helpful to at least narrow down your choices or consider solutions you hadn't thought of. At the end of the day, the real solution to caregiver burnout and fatigue is rest.

IMPACT ON OUR COGNITION

Casey shared with Caregiver Collective that, since she began caregiving, her "concentration and memory are garbage these days." She posted to the group wondering if anyone else had a similar issue. She included photos of herself standing in Target wearing slippers because she'd forgotten to put on shoes, and of burnt sandwiches in a pan because she'd forgotten to turn off the stove in the excitement of a doctor finally returning her call. She later told me that the very same night after she posted to the group, she accidentally picked up food in a drive-through without wearing any pants. Another time she forgot her house keys and had to jump over her home's fence, climb onto the second-story deck, and push in an old door. In the snow. She told me that in retrospect she finds these moments funny; she uses humor to get through. But the root of her forgetfulness is no joke—it's a cognitive ramification of stress overload:

> *People talk about how caregiving is so fulfilling and stuff....A lot of times I don't feel fulfilled, right, because you know it's a lot of work and you sometimes have to turn off your brain and be like, "We just have to do it. We just have to get through." But those funny moments, man, they get me.*

A lot of fellow caregivers described the same, that the number of things they handle simultaneously creates either brain fog or a total lapse in memory and attention to what they are doing in that moment. Cars needing to be jump-started multiple times because headlights were left on, zoning out in conversations...one person couldn't find their toaster and only later realized they'd put it in the fridge. These are instances we've all had happen at one stressful time or another (maybe not the toaster thing), but it startled me to hear just how many people noticed an uptick in forgetfulness as a result of caregiving over a period of time.

IMPACT ON OUR PHYSICAL HEALTH

Casey joked to me once: "When you're a caregiver, every day is arms day." Something we don't bring up much is the physical stress caregiving puts on our bodies. The first conversation I had with another caregiver my age was with Lea, almost a decade ago. At the time she was thirty-two, living down the street from her parents who were both chronically ill and insisted on living alone. Her dad had seizures in combination with a stroke, followed by methicillin-resistant *Staphylococcus aureus* (MRSA) in his leg that left him with a lack of mobility and coordination. Lea and her husband had become used to responding to emergency calls in the middle of the night.

"Just to kind of give you a picture, my dad is a six-foot, barrel-chested, three-hundred-pound man," Lea said. "My mom, she's a hundred and twenty pounds, five foot eight, soaking wet. If you try to put that image together of her trying to pick him up off the ground or helping him off of the toilet or getting him out of the bathtub, those are all situations that she physically just can't do anymore." I had a hard time imagining that Lea had the physical ability to bring a three-hundred-pound man to his feet, either. She filled me in on a trick she had devised, sliding her father to the nearest wall and pushing his feet against it to use as leverage. She had picked up tricks like this from other caregivers at the state-run caregiver hotline she worked for. I don't think anyone, until they're in the moment, realizes how physically demanding care work can be. More than 70 percent of caregivers reported it caused a physical strain.[19]

Millennial caregivers are more likely to experience adverse health events, such as hospitalization or an ER visit, than the general population.[20] Studies have shown that caregivers, in general, have poorer health than the rest of the population. The combination of mental and physical stress can impact our overall health and have consequences in the long run; these findings are particularly acute for caregivers our age. For example, one analysis reported that half of all caregivers surveyed used food as a coping mechanism for their stress; Millennial caregivers were found to have a 74 percent higher obesity rate when compared to the general population. Our generation's overall health is poorer, and the health impacts of caregiving on our habits and coping mechanisms need to be taken seriously.

When Alexandra's mom became paralyzed from brain cancer, wheelchair assists, such as to and from bed, were necessary and often. People had recommended mechanical lifts for Alex and her stepdad, but they didn't want the machinery in the home; they wanted her mom's life to be as peaceful as possible. But Alex knew that if she wasn't physically able to lift her mom, there was no one else there to do it. "It was one of the most physically demanding things I've ever done... All the lifting and everything, it was physically hard, and I was like, we need a lot of energy to get through this. And like mental energy, to get through the insurance and the doctors and all of that."

LET'S PULL BACK FOR A MOMENT TO CONSIDER THE MENTAL AND PHYSIcal stress caregiving has on our minds and bodies and put it into a larger context. It has been well established that, for caregivers, stress results in poorer mental and physical health and increased risk of mortality—it's no different for Millennial caregivers.[21] Millennials in general are already in poorer physical and mental health than older generations. The economy plays some role: when money is tight, you may make poorer health choices, such as eating cheaper, less nutritious foods and evading doctor bills by just not going to the doctor. Those of us who entered the workforce during a recession will face decreased life expectancy by the time we're in our forties and fifties; this poorer health is driven by behaviors (and stress coping mechanisms) like smoking, drinking, and drug overdoses.[22]

When surveyed, more Millennial caregivers reported being in poor or fair health in 2020 than in 2015.[23] Imagine a capable, busy person in their twenties or thirties (or early forties) considering their own health and checking the box that says "Poor or Fair." *This* is why caregiving is largely regarded as a public health issue, why it's important we don't just swallow our stress in its many manifestations but address it head-on.

CHAPTER 13

WE'RE FEELING *GUILTY*

"**I** FOUND THAT GUILT AND THE SHAME AROUND ALL OF IT TO BE ONE of the most surprising things," one caregiver told me. She was in her early thirties and had upended her life (where she lived, who she lived with, her relationship) to be her mom's live-in caregiver for the final months of her mother's life. The experience was grueling, physically and emotionally, as she watched her mom's health deteriorate over months. So, why the guilt and shame?

> *Why am I so resentful of this? I felt guilty about how unhappy I was [during caregiving]. My mom took care of me for seventeen years and did a fantastic, selfless job. So the fact that I was so unraveled by taking care of her for fourteen months really made me feel guilty.*

Guilty is the word I most often hear caregivers our age describe themselves as feeling. Reasons run the gamut.

> *There was a point in time, too, in my thought process where I thought, you know, if I do this, though, like, if I give up this kidney, I will have literally done everything I can. Like, the fullest degree. And I will have no guilt. I can give this kidney, then I can move to Singapore and I can feel like I've done everything.*

That's Michelle telling me how she considered donating a kidney to her mother. Before the idea of organ donation came up, Michelle had already, objectively, donated much of her life to her mom's care: in her early thirties she still lived with her parents; she'd passed on a job relocation to Singapore in order to remain at home; she battled exhaustion and struggled to have an identity outside of caregiving. Her social life was way on the back burner: she either didn't have the time, or the energy, or she felt guilty taking a moment for herself. Michelle gave a lot of herself and, maybe, more than most. Still, she felt like she was supposed to give *more*. That it was her responsibility. On many levels, she felt no one else could provide for her mom's health like she could; it's a narrative that had taken root decades earlier.

When Michelle first learned from doctors that a living kidney donation was her mother's best chance for improvement, she took the blood test thinking it was unlikely she'd be a viable candidate. She was a match. Her parents were clear they did not want Michelle to go through with the donation, but that didn't deter her.

Was she comfortable donating her kidney? She wasn't sure. She turned to networks of living kidney donors who had already gone through the process and were willing to speak with her one-on-one. Michelle was affirmed by hearing they were fine, able to have children, leading happy and productive lives. Then she found a Facebook group for kidney donors who were struggling with negative health repercussions from the decision, and they offered a different perspective. Michelle weighed the factors: she was an only child; her relatives were all older; if something went wrong, she wondered, who would take care of her?

She went through what she called the "huge battery of tests" and screenings required for a living donor candidate to move forward in the process. It was the mandatory psych evaluation that had the most impact on her ultimate decision.

"There's this sense of, if you gave up your organ, and this person who received it then didn't take care of themselves, how would you react? Would you then become more resentful? I don't know if I would be able to live with that sort of resentment if it didn't go well." Considering that in the past, her mom had resisted taking medications and managing her diabetes, Michelle wasn't necessarily convinced her mother would take the new kidney as a fresh start to take better care of her health. And Michelle would be there watching it all, knowing that her sacrifice was taken for granted; not by her mother directly, but through her actions... and that's if the surgery was a success. There was also the chance that, after the transplant, the donated kidney would fail. It was a lot for Michelle to consider. She thought about what was driving her to donate in the first place, and ultimately decided not to go through with it.

At the end of the day, I realized that I was wanting to do it to be rid of the guilt. I don't think it was hard to come to the realization that "I don't think I want to." And at the same time, that's kind of okay, to not want to give up your organ.

I just want to let that sit there for a moment. Michelle's self-affirmation was "It's okay to not want to give up your organ." From an outside perspective, it's easy to tell Michelle not to be so hard on herself. Caregiving does not require replacing the organs of the person you care for with your own body. Many people wouldn't have taken the initial blood test in the first place. I also know a lot of caregivers reading this would have considered the same and thrown themselves into that fire. No one asked Michelle to do this (in fact, her parents had discouraged it), but Michelle had set a very high bar for herself to live up to. The cultural expectation of devotion to family was instilled by her upbringing, she said, but the levels to which she held herself accountable were her own doing. She had, you could argue, unreasonably high expectations of herself, as a daughter and as a caregiver, that she felt guilty if she didn't uphold.

WE'RE GOOD AT FEELING GUILTY

Caregivers, I notice, often confuse care or devotion with martyrdom. It's an impulse, even if the idea is quickly dismissed.

Millennials feel guilt when we believe high expectations (ours or someone else's) haven't been met. We don't want to disappoint, possibly because while growing up our parents had high expectations of us. This plays out in our adult behavior. In a *Huffington Post* article, a group of therapists were asked what they hear Millennials bring up the most in therapy.[1] High on the list: saying no to other people, especially parents. "Millennials are overeager to impress and have a deep sense of guilt when they say no," the article stated. A study by the Thriving Center of Psychology found more than half of Millennials surveyed had a hard time saying no to someone else (the only generation who found it harder: Gen Z).[2]

Millennials have the most trouble setting boundaries with family.[3] The people they struggle the most with saying no to include parents (especially Mom), friends, their partner, and their boss. (See the overlap with whom caregivers are struggling to balance and please?) We feel guilty when we can't, or don't want to, fulfill someone else's expectations of us. We've transferred our parents' high expectations of us onto ourselves. Remember how Millennials struggle with perfectionism? Expectations we hold ourselves to can be the harshest, and to "say no" to their pursuit in full would create disappointment in ourselves. We'd think we didn't do enough, that we could've done more. For caregivers, the stakes are the health and well-being, even the life, of someone we love. We feel guilty if we don't throw everything we've got at it.

WE'RE OVERDOING IT

A *Forbes* article from 2019 states that 66 percent of Millennials are workaholics.[4] We were the first totally connected generation, with the internet at our fingertips. To prove ourselves and keep our jobs, we internalized the idea that we should be working all the time, and our phones mean the office can always reach us.[5] We work martyrs felt guilty taking days off, wanting instead to prove we were completely dedicated to the role. There was always something more we could be doing, and when we don't accomplish tasks (even menial ones), it's followed by guilt for not completing them. This all led to what's referred to as *Millennial burnout.*

In recent years, our priorities shifted dramatically: now Millennials are the generation that cares most about work-life balance.[6] But that doesn't mean we're taking it easy: the "life" part may include running an Etsy shop or training for a marathon.[7] We've taken our learned workaholic tendencies and sprinkled them onto our private lives and personal decision-making...and our caregiving. Even when you're taking a break, there's still something that can be done: try that doctor's office again, google the latest symptom you noticed.

"I think there's a tendency to do everything you can until you can't," Michelle said. "Like, 'Just do it. It's your loved one,' right?...A huge part of it is the mental load. You're always on and trying to think of better ways to do things, and sometimes you can get lost in feeling that's not enough." Michelle passed some responsibilities off to her dad and learned to stand back, trust he would handle them. Still, she said, "it took getting comfortable with that idea of feeling guilty."

The idea that we're not living up to what's expected of us, even if that was something we defined ourselves and projected onto the person we care for, is a massive disappointment we do everything to avoid.

GUILT FOR PUTTING YOURSELF FIRST

Think about Michelle, who was ready to sacrifice her own organs. It was guilt, Michelle explicitly stated, that drove her to consider kidney donation. Then, after deciding against it, she felt guilty for not going through with it.

"You read all these posts of people who did [donate their kidney] and they're like, 'I would do it again in a heartbeat.' And then you feel so shady about yourself because they're like, 'That's my dad. That's my mom.'" The implication was, *it's my parent, so I will do anything for them*—and Michelle hadn't. "That's been a whole other kind of journey," she said. It's impossible to compare yourself; also, as a general rule: don't compare yourself. But Michelle's guilt was less about other people and more that, in a rare moment, she had chosen to put herself first. "I could help her in all of this and, not only am I not choosing to, I'm doing it because technically it's in *my* best interest. That's kind of hard to come to terms with. And I think it's hard to feel okay with it, even though it is [okay]." Ultimately, Michelle's decision was an exercise in setting a boundary for herself.

CONFLICT AROUND SETTING BOUNDARIES

Like saying no, boundary setting is something Millennials struggle with.[8] (Although, since the pandemic and remote work blurred the lines between our jobs and our personal lives, Millennials have become better about boundary setting at work to achieve a better work-life balance.[9]) While in our minds we may have an idea of what we are cool with doing (and what we are not), voicing and upholding these boundaries in our relationships is another thing…doing so can press on our "guilty nerve."

"When you start caregiving, it becomes this weird codependence," Kaci said. "That's something I struggle a lot with and have to go to therapy for, is learning how to set boundaries and not feel intense amounts of guilt if I say no." Kaci brings up a really important point: codependence. The belief that our loved one cannot survive, or survive well, without us. Codependence can be exerted by the person being cared for, and can arise for a host of reasons: feeling helpless because a physical or mental impairment means they have a hard time getting up to go to the bathroom or they need you to go to the store for their medication; feeling lonely and relying on you for company; or maybe they don't speak English well and rely on you to translate in the course of daily needs or pharmacy runs or doctor appointments or all of it. Maybe it's all these reasons.

I also notice a codependent attachment can be created on the side of the caregiver. I think I did this out of fear my dad could be gone, a prospect that terrified me. If he was in my sights, he was here. There is also this binding of your life to their care because you think, *If I don't handle this myself, it won't get done. Or it won't be done the right way. If I'm not there for them, no one else will be.*

"That level of responsibility that people feel can make it harder for somebody to set those boundaries," Christina Irving said. "Because then [if something bad happens] they take on that guilt of 'I could have prevented this thing from happening.' And you don't necessarily know that that's true."

I believed that my momentary absence would create a familial void no one else could fill in the same way; sure, an aide could sit with my dad through his dinner, but I was *his daughter.* The prospect of the void I'd create obliterated my personal boundaries, and I acted in service of what I thought would make my dad happy or what I felt he needed.

Laura, who cared for her dad alongside her brother, named a different reason for the attachment they both had to their dad through his illnesses. "Both of us feel a little bit like we really tried to live Dad's life for him, in a way, at the end with the Alzheimer's. And it detracted from life, really. He'd be shocked or mortified to hear that, because that's the thing he wanted least was to be a burden." In retrospect, she thinks it may have been too much.

Therapy helped Michelle identify where she needed to set boundaries with her parents and, even more difficult, to act on them. Therapy showed her that she can make decisions for herself, and although it feels hard, it's okay to do. It has also helped Michelle sift through where caregiving ended and her own identity began. Moving out into her own apartment was a major step in setting a limit between her mom's illness and care and Michelle's own life. Michelle's decision to move out wasn't binary, a choice between herself and her mom. She was able to figure out how to carve out space for her own needs while continuing to help her mom. It just looked different now...and so did Michelle's guilt.

"Now that I have moved out...I think I might have swung too far in this [direction]. Now I feel like, I don't know...my dad's part of this caregiving partnership, too, so I'm just trying to figure out how I can help [to] make sure he's not in it alone, too overwhelmed." I think this new wave of guilt, that's she's left her dad holding the bag, is a natural reaction to stepping back from handling everything. With less on her plate, she thinks she's not doing enough. Despite that, "It's been a really positive change." (For therapist Christina Irving's advice on setting boundaries, flip back to Chapter 5.)

"DID I MAKE THE RIGHT DECISION?"

Caregivers encounter a gauntlet of difficult decisions, and it can be easy to obsess over what the outcome would have been if you'd chosen another way—especially when, maybe, it would've benefited the person you care for. I often notice this regarding medical decisions.

When it came to choosing whether to put their dad on hospice care or not, Laura and her brother weighed the decision carefully. It was a mental back-and-forth. She knows they made the best decision with the information they had, but when we talked about it over a year later, I noticed even the discussion put her right back in the throes of weighing the options with uncertainty. Second-guessing is a form of anxiety. When you're caregiving, the idea that you chose wrong, and the person's health or happiness is affected, induces more guilt.

Moving your family member to a living facility can also be a massive source of guilt; often I think it's the guilt itself that makes the decision so difficult. One caregiver expressed what she called "survivor's guilt" for doing fun things while her mother is "stuck" in a nursing home. Another said her father is in an assisted living facility, and she struggles with guilt over it daily.

Erin cared for her mom at home for five years until her mother's terminal illness and needs progressed and Erin could no longer manage it. Her mother moved to a nursing home, and Erin feels guilty that she's unhappy living there. The disapproval some family members have expressed to Erin, complaining about the facility, makes her feel even worse. She knows it was the only viable decision to make for her mom's care but regrets that she doesn't have the money or a large home to continue caring for her mom herself.

Christina Irving says the pressure we put on ourselves to do everything perfectly is a setup for guilty feelings. If your job is to take care of your family member and things don't go the way you hoped, or something bad happens, it doesn't mean you didn't do your job well.

"That, I think, is an unrealistic expectation that a lot of caregivers put on themselves and it's understandable," Irving said. "But it often sets people up for failure or sets people up for a feeling like they have to invest all of themselves into that caregiving role. And that's just not realistic for people both with time and energy and someone's own health and well-being." She advises caregivers to "come to terms with that for themselves" by realizing there are things you'd like to do, or wish you could, that are not possible. It's also important to give yourself permission to set boundaries to take care of yourself.

GUILT FOR OUR OWN FEELINGS

I feel guilty for thinking this is hard when I'm the healthy one. What they're dealing with is so much worse. Do these thoughts sound familiar? Often we compare our feelings to the experience of the person we care for, which leads us to feel guilty for having feelings at all. We shame ourselves for our own emotional distress within the experience.

Debbie found she compared her emotional responses with her mom to how a "perfect" version of herself would handle things. If she didn't live up to that high standard, her testy reactions to stressful moments with her mom led to feelings of guilt. A professional therapist, she recognizes some of their stressful interactions follow patterns; she knows techniques to manage them, but acting on that is not always realistic:

> We [therapists] get angry and frustrated and discouraged as well, like anyone else. Sometimes I create my own expectation and pressure on myself because I have this [professional] background. I'll have moments where I

think, "Well, you should know how to handle this." Really being hard on myself to feel like I need to do better, or I need to manage my own reactions better.

It's a lot of pressure to put on yourself, to hold yourself to a higher standard than others, but there are those high expectations again. Debbie's learned to manage expectations for her own behavior in what can be a stressful role...and, critical for caregivers, to have compassion for herself. Now her self-talk is this:

"You're gonna make mistakes. You're gonna have times where you don't handle things as well as you want to, just like everybody else, and it doesn't matter that this is your profession." So it's more about, can you just be nicer to yourself? Forgive yourself for not being perfect at the standard that you think you should be.

LET GO OF HIGHEST EXPECTATIONS AND PERFECTION

I admittedly am, at most times, a perfectionist, so I understand the irony of my proselytizing this advice, but: let go of perfection. Caregiving and someone else's emotional or physical state is out of your complete control; perfection is an ideal, not a reality. I'm not saying give up—far from it. But I am advising you to manage your expectations when it comes to what you are willing to give and your own limitations.

Sometimes—maybe a lot of times—you'll make mistakes. Alexandra, who moved home to care for her mom with brain cancer, didn't realize at the time how much she was blaming herself:

There was rage, but I don't think I expected so much guilt and shame...constantly feeling like you're doing things wrong. It was actually when I worked with some woo-woo energy healer that I finally said to someone, out loud for the first time ever, that my mom fell out of her wheelchair once when I was walking with her. And I realized how much I had carried the guilt of her falling out. And, to this day, I sometimes question some of the decisions I made, but I think I found a little more compassion for: I did the best I could with the knowledge I had at the time.

One of Laura's dad's doctors told her that caregiving is making decisions in the fog of war. You can come up with the perfect plan, but don't assume you'll get to use it. At a certain point, survival, as Laura kept describing it, has to be good enough.

Michelle, who, in this chapter alone, has come a long way, has words of wisdom here:

There's this phrase that I have found myself telling my mom and I think it's super important: It doesn't have to be perfect to be good. In this role, where you can't really control everything, you can't plan for anything try as you might, being able to go with the flow and be[ing] okay with it not matching necessarily that initial expectation that you have are super important because I think it'll set you up for less disappointment.

CHAPTER 14

WE'RE FEELING *TERRIFIED* AND *TRAUMATIZED*

A FEW YEARS AGO, MY MOM ASKED ME TO PICK HER UP FROM A ROUTINE colonoscopy. When I arrived to the outpatient facility, I was met by a nurse who informed me that my mom was fine and waiting for me to take her home. Nevertheless, as I approached the recovery room, panic crept in. My breathing thinned, my vision clouded, a deep fog settled over my brain. I stepped through the curtain to her bed, and the rhythmic heart monitor beeps triggered acute sensory flashbacks to a few years earlier—the unexpected hospital visits I rushed to, each time arriving terrified of the condition I'd find my father in; the final week spent in the hospital during what unfolded to be the end of his life. Those mechanical monitor beeps…the thin hospital blanket my mom was waiting under, smiling from anesthesia and a passing health grade…they put me right back there. Woozy, I grabbed for a chair.

I didn't know at the time that I was having an episode of PTSD.

This isn't rhetoric; after years of caregiving, I was diagnosed by my therapist as showing symptoms of post-traumatic stress disorder. After my dad passed, classic PTSD symptoms, which included intrusive flashbacks, being dazed when distressed, and avoiding medical settings reminiscent of his disease, recurred. (These are also symptoms of acute stress disorder, or ASD, a potential precursor to PTSD experienced during and up to four weeks after a traumatic event.[1] PTSD occurs in the period after.)

At the time, PTSD as a result of caregiving wasn't something talked about, even among researchers or caregivers themselves, but I knew my response couldn't be a one-off. The article I wrote about it for the *Washington Post* received a wave of responses from caregivers of all ages, who had experiences similar to mine and suspected PTSD but hadn't addressed it by name. Most had associated PTSD with veterans and didn't want the indirect comparison to be viewed as undue exaggeration, but in refraining from using the term they didn't validate the possibility that their own caregiving experience could be considered clinically traumatic. They didn't know that it is. And it is.

The American Psychiatric Association defines PTSD as "a psychiatric disorder that may occur in people who have experienced or witnessed a traumatic event, series of events, or set of circumstances."[2] It presents as "intense, disturbing thoughts and feelings" related to that trauma that continue to occur long after the event has ended. For caregivers, an acute event may be a phone call informing you a loved one is in the hospital or the doctor visit when you first received a terrible diagnosis. It can be the result of being bedside in the hospital or witnessing jarring medical procedures performed on a person you love. In some cases, caregiving itself, particularly caregiving over a long period of time, can be considered the traumatic "set of circumstances" the APA refers to.

Although more research is needed to truly understand the issue, existing studies support that caregiving can put people at risk of PTSD. Research conducted on family members of ICU patients at both the University of California, San Francisco, and Samuel Merritt University in Oakland, California, found high rates of PTSD symptoms in those considered "decision-makers" (35 percent and 42 percent, respectively).[3] The ICU event itself can be triggering for caregivers: sights and sounds experienced there, as well as the uncertainty and severity of the situation, may be relived through distressing flashbacks even months later.[4] Family members of patients were found to experience acute stress disorder as early as arrival in the ICU; their ASD "score" at that time was equivalent to that of someone admitted to a PTSD unit for psychiatric treatment.[5] Another study of caregivers with family in the ICU found that their ASD and PTSD rates remained relatively stable from hospital admission to six months post-hospitalization, suggesting discharge does not alleviate the emotional trauma.[6] Although acute and post-traumatic stress symptoms may remain invisible or unknown to people in the life of the caregiver, the experience and its intensity should not be undermined.

Just to be clear, I want to underline: PTSD is a condition resulting from someone's own experience and what they've witnessed or lived through as a caregiver. When researchers studied family caregivers of people in palliative care, when their imminent passing was not an unexpected event, caregiver trauma was found to be separate from the perceived suffering of the patient.[7] It is rooted in the caregiver's experience and does not end when the suffering of their loved one does.

PSYCHOLOGY TODAY DOES A GREAT JOB OF BREAKING DOWN PTSD SYMPtoms into three categories: re-experiencing, avoidance, and hyperarousal:[8]

RE-EXPERIENCING

Re-experiencing includes flashbacks; it's how we often see presentations of PTSD in the movies. The memories are disruptive and come on suddenly, quick flashes in which you may not "see" anything, but your body and mind are back in that space. Re-experiencing can also occur through nightmares or bad dreams related to the original trauma. It can include frightening projecting thoughts of terrible things that might happen, and turning over in your mind potential reactions of what you will do when it does.

AVOIDANCE

Avoidance is what the body and mind do (consciously or subconsciously) to protect you against feeling the pain and fear of trauma again. It doesn't work. Avoidance can lead you to feeling frozen or numb inside; it even accounts for blurred vision and brain fog. According to my therapist, the body can shut down—go into sleep mode, effectively—to protect you from taking in what your subconscious mind perceives as emotionally dangerous. Avoiding places, objects, or events that remind you of the event is a hallmark sign. The memory problems we hear caregivers talk about? That can also be a form of avoidance related to acute or post-traumatic stress. Symptoms also include feeling guilty, depressed, or worried all the time and losing interest in activities you enjoyed before. The really unhealthy thing about avoidance is that it prevents us from addressing our pain and fear, which is necessary to manage or overcome our stress symptoms.

Numbness can also be a sign of *desensitization*, another coping response to repeated trauma. When you deal with something traumatic often, like trips to the ER, they begin to feel normal; our minds don't recognize we are continuing to cope with trauma, but that doesn't stop the effects of trauma from building. One caregiver told me how each trip to the hospital used to feel devastating but they have become so common that her internal response now is "Well, here we go again."

HYPERAROUSAL

Hyperarousal is another symptom we hear caregivers bring up often. It's that sense of always being on high alert or, as *Psychology Today* describes it, "hypervigilance from being in a state of chronic stress, coupled with responsibility to monitor another person's safety or critical needs."[9] Maybe a caregiver has experienced a rainfall of "other shoes" dropping, or maybe the other shoe dropped with such a thud it left a crack in the floor. Maybe it's just the idea of shoes dropping and we're not gonna see it coming—any of these scenarios leave us constantly searching the sky for those fucking shoes. But it's not just big things we're on the lookout for, it's…everything. Hyperarousal from PTSD can mean our minds never rest from assessing potential threats and it's exhausting. The person experiencing PTSD may be easily startled by noises or have trouble falling asleep. It explains why hyperarousal can also be experienced as feeling irritable, tense, sore, or having angry outbursts.

MILITARY CAREGIVERS MAY EXPERIENCE A DIFFERENT DISORDER, known as secondary traumatic stress (STS). STS presents very similarly to PTSD (the same symptoms) but is the result of indirect trauma: by empathizing with their loved one who experienced the trauma (such as a soldier who lost their leg after stepping on a mine), the family member can "take on the traumatized person's feelings, experiences and memories as their own."[10] Essentially, by imagining the traumatic event lived by their loved one, even filling in any blanks on their own to "relive" the moment and put themselves in the other person's shoes, they themselves indirectly absorb the trauma…and its emotional aftermath. The Wounded Warrior Project shares that the family member with STS may also adopt the same coping mechanisms their care recipient uses (such as avoidance) to avoid an episode or behavioral breakdown from their loved one.[11] They warn a doubling-down of negative coping mechanisms may ultimately serve to exacerbate the problem.

AT THE TIME, I DIDN'T REALIZE THAT I WAS EXPERIENCING SYMPTOMS OF PTSD. I also didn't realize I was a prime candidate: a "younger" caregiver, female, and the family member involved in decision-making for my dad. The fact that he was my parent and we had a close relationship is also considered a risk factor.[12] Time spent at his bedside in the ICU, it seemed, sealed the deal with jarring images, the fear and panic I felt.

A long period of caregiving can also mean increased risk for PTSD; caregiving over an extended period of time produces psychological stress found to be consistent with a chronic stress experience.[13] Kaci has been caring for her mother, in various ways, for years. She's been diagnosed with complex PTSD (C-PTSD), which can result from "prolonged or repeated trauma over months or years."[14]

"I think a lot of it has to do with when my dad had passed, when I was younger. I have a lot of fear that this just compounded. I think there's things that will, like, trigger a response [in] me, one of them definitely is my mom's health." Kaci's mom has cardiovascular disease; she had her first surgery to treat it when Kaci was ten years old. Since then, she's had a series of strokes and a series of surgeries, some planned and others performed in emergencies.

"When I was twenty-five, right before I left for Europe [to work as an au pair], that's when my mom had the emergency surgery. She knew her health was failing, and she had a suicide attempt. I had to go through a lot when I was twenty-five, because my mom was severely depressed. She had been depressed since my dad had died but hadn't really, I don't think, ever really processed it either." I mentioned to Kaci a correlation between ICU stays and caregiver PTSD; she told me that after an emergency surgery, her mom spent four months in the ICU. "They thought she was gonna die. I woke up in the middle of the night and spent the night on the floor. That is where, like, a lot of my PTSD comes from." Years later, each time her mother tells Kaci something hurts that is reminiscent of that time, Kaci is triggered into thinking she will have to live through that all over again.

Kaci is like a checklist for PTSD risk factors: young, female, close relation to the care recipient, ICU stays, caregiving over an extended period of time, on and on and on. But someone doesn't need to check all these boxes to experience caregiving as a trauma and to live with the emotional fallout for years to come.

"THERE'S THE GRIEF OF LOSING YOUR PARENT AND THEN THERE'S, FOR me, there was the trauma of caretaking," Alexandra said, explaining the feelings she's had since her mother passed. "I didn't realize that those were actually two separate things, that I needed to give care and attention to both to kind of heal from. Because one was about my mom and losing all the thirty to thirty-five years I thought I was going to have with her and missing her every now and then; the other one is everything I went through in that fourteen months [as her primary caregiver]." Alex's mom, you remember, had brain cancer, and Alex left her life living and working abroad to move into her mom's upstate New York home and care for her. Like me, it was after her parent died that she fully recognized caregiving and her mom's illness as traumatic experiences she needed to do healing work on. I asked her if, at the time, she was aware of the situation being a trauma.

"In those last couple of months there were moments where I called my dad crying, like saying: I don't... I don't know what to do. I feel like I can't put mom in the hospital, but, I said, I'm kind of like fantasizing about being in a small car accident because I want to go to the hospital. I was, we were all, tapped out mentally, physically, everything. So I was very aware. It was not a mystery to me that I was not okay." Her fantasy of getting hit by a car was not about wanting to get hurt, she said. She just wanted a break. For someone to take care of her.

Alex told me that although she was aware of the trauma she was experiencing, she did little in the moment in the way of self-care to help herself; but she did try to get back to work. At the time, she was "reaching her breaking point" and needed a little bit of her own life back. Interestingly, research suggests that the impulse to go back to work may actually help reduce potential PTSD symptoms; while work is a stressor for caregivers, it can also provide respite and social and financial support that can aid our well-being in these intense moments.[15]

FEAR

Intense fear is one of the signs of acute stress disorder.[16] Fear can affect our well-being, our decision-making, and in moments can hit so strong it feels paralyzing. It was only after caregiving that I realized, after years in anticipation of the other shoe dropping, I'd adopted a fear that trickled into all areas of my life: fear of making the wrong decision, fear the worst could happen at any moment. My father's illness was the first time in my life I'd seen a consequence play out as death; I'm certain that experiencing this harsh reality early in adulthood instilled a previously foreign sense of caution and trepidation my peers didn't seem to have.

Debbie told me about the fear she felt when her mom was still living alone, before she moved into assisted living. Each time the phone rang was a scare of a potential crisis. I've already noted how phone calls can be a major stress trigger for caregivers, but they can also strike a pang of fear. It took quite a while after my dad passed for me to turn off my phone's ringer at night, because: *what IF*. Being temporarily unreachable wasn't a luxury I was used to; calls from unknown numbers still induced a panic response.

"When you're living with that 'waiting for the other shoe to drop' sort of feeling, it can take away the ability to enjoy a lot of things," Debbie said. "In this last year especially, and since moving my mom to assisted living, I've realized how much I really just need to take life less seriously and learn to have more fun again. So I'm kind of in the process of doing that for myself." She said seeing a therapist has helped reduce some of her anxiety around fear.

IF YOU HAD TOLD ME WHEN MY FATHER GOT ILL THAT I COULD BE AT RISK of developing PTSD as a result of caring for him, my response probably would've been, "I'll be fine." Like Alex, I brushed aside any distress—such as panicking when my phone rang with an unknown number—as typical because why *wouldn't* this be upsetting? Caregivers often normalize negative responses, not realizing something deeper is at play. Making matters worse, they often delay their own mental health treatment to prioritize others' care.[17]

Dr. Ranak Trivedi, a clinical and health psychologist and researcher at Stanford University who specializes in military veteran and caregiver research, advises about the importance of being attuned to your thoughts and emotions. "One thing to really watch for, are you able to disconnect from the care recipient's experience?" If the person you care for is in a safe space, do you still perceive potential danger and that you're the only one responsible? These thoughts, she said, would be indicative of hyperarousal. She recommends recognizing that you are overestimating threat in the environment. Coming to this awareness yourself, or having someone you trust point out this behavior, allows you to cognitively restructure your thoughts.

Dr. Trivedi recommends asking yourself, "What is the worst that can happen? What are the chances that that's going to happen? And what am I giving up by not taking this low risk, [such as] stepping out of the house?" Then experiment with taking a step back. She also stresses having self-compassion when judging your own thoughts. "Talking to ourselves, reasoning using real words…like, 'I know I'm feeling this way because I'm worried'" can reframe our thinking. In the case of intrusive flashbacks, she says mindfulness through anchoring exercises, such as labeling five nearby objects or colors, can root you in the present and allow those flashbacks to diminish. Exercises like this remind you that you are in control of your own thinking.

Retraumatization, like how Kaci compounds fear for her mom's present-day health concerns with previous experiences, is "like experiencing double the stress in the moment," Dr. Trivedi said. You are experiencing the distress of high-level care while reminded of an unprocessed trauma.

"To the extent people have the capacity at the time, challenge your own thoughts to say, 'This is different. This is a new experience. It might have the same ending, but it's not the same journey.' Those reminders, that there's a separation of time that has happened, can be really effective." The ideal treatment, she said, is undergoing professional therapy. Some studies have been done on potential interventions healthcare providers can conduct to address caregiver PTSD and mental health; we'll talk about them in a later chapter.

TRAUMA ACTIVISM AS CATHARSIS AFTER CAREGIVING

Advocacy is, in some instances, a mechanism for coping with past trauma. Some caregivers, like me, start support groups or advocate for caregiver rights...some victims of gun violence push publicly for stricter gun laws...some who've experienced domestic violence go on to careers in law. We've seen this often in our country, particularly in the last decade. According to therapists specializing in grief and trauma, activism serves a host of functions for the bereaved, including helping to find meaning in senseless personal loss and acting as an outlet for engagement. It can be a way to help others in ways you wish you could have received help, to take power over an event that was anything but in your control. Some people find deep healing in activism. And on some levels, I have. But it's also my experience that speaking publicly for the sake of advocacy can painfully evoke PTS symptoms.

When I wrote my first piece on caregiving for *Cosmo*, a friend said, "Writing that must have felt so cathartic for you." Not really. Writing it was fucking painful: In my mind I was reliving some of the saddest things I've witnessed and experienced and it felt like reopening a deep wound of loss. I sat there typing with tears pouring down my face, and not in a soul-cleansing way but with profound grief that remains at the ready. Am I glad it gets the message out? Yes. That's why I was doing it. But getting there, the process, does not yet feel good. It feels like I want ice cream.

Some research suggests that people recover from traumas faster if they can simply talk about them, but talking about grief repeatedly or with people who don't understand may not be helpful.

This isn't something our culture talks about often, but it's important to consider—particularly for an activist generation like ours. I notice some caregivers in my group who jump into advocacy action in the immediate aftermath of their loved one's death, and I wonder if they've had time to process the big event that just happened or the entire experience that led up to it. I think often that when caregiving ends, it leaves a void we look to fill in order to, somehow, continue caregiving. To still feel connected to the role and, more potently, to the person who is no longer there. I warn them, give it a minute—not in connecting with others about their experience but in publicly engaging by regularly repeating painful stories or details.

As much as I implore my generation to share their care experiences to build awareness, I'm personally aware of the emotional toll this can take; I caution people to set their own boundaries in what they share, and how. When dealing with caregiver trauma, crossing the line between catharsis and reliving trauma prolongs our healing.

CHAPTER 15

WE'RE FEELING *GRIEF*

A FRIEND ONCE TOLD ME THAT GRIEF IS LIKE PLAYING THE PIANO: FROM one day to the next you don't know which key will get played or in what order. One day you see a funny movie and find yourself laughing with abandon, the next day you can't get out of bed. After my dad passed, I experienced shock at ever having lived with his illness at all, that my dad was ever sick. But, if I'm honest, I'd also already been grieving for years.

Grief is often associated with bereavement, but caregivers experience grief much earlier. The first traces may appear the day we hear a painful diagnosis; it continues in varying shapes as long as we are caregiving. Often we don't understand what we're feeling or how to identify it; the plaguing void of loss at the back of your heart's chamber can be confusing when the person is still alive. You may be overcome by the ways in which the person is no longer active in your life. Though my dad's disease didn't alter his personality, it did make speaking much more arduous for him. Conversation would last the same length of time but became limited as he took longer to articulate what he wanted to say; the words took strength for him to vocalize. I mourned his input that I knew I wasn't getting or asking for, which had always been instrumental and subversively funny and comforting for me, whether I took his advice or not. The sadness was a feeling I had but a thought I suppressed. The guy was still here, *be grateful*. And I was. I talked myself out of the sadder thoughts; I didn't allow myself to dwell and pushed through. (I have just given you a nice example of avoidance.)

In other moments you may not be able to help thinking ahead to what the hell you'll do after they're gone, then feel guilty for having these thoughts and share them with no one. In a way, having these secret thoughts about life without the person feels like going behind their back. It's a massive energy suck that can knock you out or build to a breaking point that is then expressed in toxic ways.

THE BURDEN OF GRIEF

One NIH paper I read states that ongoing family caregiving not only involves the "burden of caregiving" but also the "burden of grief" as the caregiver struggles to reconcile "who the person was," "who they are now," and "who they will become."[1] Unlike in a divorce, where the relationship ends, in caregiving, the person changes, but the relationship continues—although changed, driven by the person's condition. Because the relationship remains present but requires modification, the grief experienced by the caregiver needs to be managed differently from the grief of someone in bereavement.[2]

For a lot of us, "who they are now" is shaped by diseases or events that result in cognitive changes, like Parkinson's, Alzheimer's, traumatic brain injury, mental illness, or a stroke. Communication, behavior, and memory may be changed, or regularly fluctuating, and in some instances the person's personality changes as well. When personality or behavior greatly changes but the person's physical body remains intact, the mind-fuck of it wreaks havoc on the caregiver and can negatively affect their mental and physical health.[3]

People who find themselves caregiving young don't just grieve the person who has changed; like we've already touched on, they also mourn the lives they thought they'd have, the milestones that have been compromised or, they fear, missed entirely. In cases when the cared-for person ultimately passes, some caregivers grieve the loss of the role they took on intimately and intensely for all that time. Members of Caregiver Collective have described their ongoing grief as an "emotional roller coaster" that gets set into motion not once in the process, like a sudden death might, but each time there is a new symptom or display of decline. More time spent caregiving can result in heightened grief, both of the anticipatory variety and in bereavement.[4]

Caregivers are grieving, and it is completely normal. But, unaddressed, grief plays out in our lives in a variety of negative ways: it can, frankly, lead us into depression.[5] It can cause us to socially isolate even more from the people in our life and impact our relationships. It can lead to a sense of hopelessness or helplessness. It can create uncertainty about our own identity.

We may not recognize the sadness we feel as grief, so it goes unidentified and we push it aside, carrying on with our days in spite of the weight and confusion of it all. According to experts, naming the feelings can make them easier to cope with, so we're going to do just that. Let's unpack the various types of grief associated with caregiving and *what*, exactly, young caregivers can do about it.

AMBIGUOUS LOSS FOR THE PERSON

My mom doesn't remember many things anymore, so she didn't remember it was my birthday. I wouldn't have expected her to at this point in her illness. It was a very rough day for her, where she was just very enraged, very dysregulated. And I think as much as I've had to do a lot of my own sort of coaching and therapy and supporting myself, it's moments like that where a sad inner child is like, I wish my parents would be able to be emotionally present for me. I don't expect anything big from my mom, I would just like for us to have a nice interaction. And unfortunately, we weren't able to have that [on] that day.

Debbie just wanted to spend her birthday with her mom; but now Debbie's mom didn't know what day it was. Logically, Debbie understood, but emotionally she was hurt. She missed her mom, who she was before dementia, and mourned what she missed from their relationship. This is *ambiguous loss.*

Ambiguous loss is what you might feel when a loved one is physically present, but not emotionally or mentally available.[6] It's a response to "psychological absence," or witnessing the person's decline over time. Debbie told me that she didn't realize what she was feeling in that moment on her birthday; it wasn't until she was sitting with her husband later that she realized she was hurt and had an emotional need that her mother, on that day, was not able to meet:

> It's hard to watch the slow loss of functioning in the person that you care about. It's just like this ever-moving process. There's points where I'm like, "Okay, I've accepted that this is where we are," and then something changed. And then you have to ask [of] yourself the same thing again, like, "Okay, I'm going to try my best to accept what's happening at this juncture."

The contrast between who the person is today and their "old" self can cause complications in a caregiver's grief and make the loss gain significance over time.[7] Memories of the "old" self live alongside accepting and adjusting to the "new" person. It can be difficult to process.

Alexandra's mom, who had brain cancer, became paralyzed and "very quickly" lost her ability to speak. When Alex moved back in to care for her, the first couple of months her mother was still lucid; Alex has happy memories of the time spent there with her, but things became more difficult as she watched her mother change:

> It was just that beautiful time of year in upstate New York and I have almost fond memories I look back on, of bringing her up to the porch and both of us just napping out there and doing these, like, spa days in the living room and kind of nice things. But it pretty quickly felt like she really wasn't there at all and it was hard to enjoy those moments.

Erica, whose mom has multiple system atrophy, misses her mom's guidance in the day-to-day. Erica's mom is only in her sixties, and Erica finds that she's already navigating life without her in ways her friends won't understand for years: "Just when you call your mom and you go, 'Oh, how much garlic do I use in that sauce recipe you used to make when I was a kid?' Or as simple as, 'Should I take this other job that they're offering me at school?' Adult decisions that you start to have to make at a certain age, you—" She began crying, upset that she now makes these decisions on her own, then apologized for the tears.

Because the person is still there physically, you might feel like you're overreacting or feel guilty for being sad when the person is still alive.[8] You might tell yourself sadness is wrong and, instead, convince yourself to be grateful they're still here. What I've come to realize while researching this: you can be both. You can be grateful they are still here, and you can be sad for the parts of them that are no longer available to you.

Christina Irving suggests expanding your thinking to include both of these realities. "It's a process of acknowledging what's lost but also trying to find the pieces that are still [rewarding]." For example, think to yourself, "'This person isn't the same person they were before and I can still have a relationship with them or enjoy certain activities with them'...It often feels like holding two contradictory thoughts in your mind at the same time." (For caregivers who mourn the person they themselves used to be before care, the same thinking can be applied.)

ONCE YOU DO IDENTIFY YOUR SADNESS, YOU MIGHT THINK THAT, BECAUSE the person is still alive, others won't understand why you're so upset. It also may be because other people don't notice the same changes in the person you do: perceptions of change that the caregiver experiences between the "old" and "new" person are subjective and may often outweigh the actual differences.[9] This can determine how we respond and cope. Debbie echoed other caregivers when she told me that there are moments she's overcome by emotions but, because of responsibilities, she doesn't have time to express them: "With caregiving, sometimes we're just on the go or there's not time to sit in your car and cry. It's just like, 'Well, we need to get to this doctor's appointment. I'm just gonna have to contain this and take it out later.' But sometimes you have to do that."

Some caregivers shared insights on what they tell themselves in the face of ambiguous loss. Jesus filmed *Care to Laugh*, a documentary about what it looks like for him to be a caregiver to his parents while pursuing his career as a stand-up comedian. At the time of filming, a few years ago now, his mother's cognition problems were evident and she had a hard time physically moving around on her own.

> *Looking back at that documentary is very hard because I know where my mom was, and it was very difficult. But looking back, I'm like, in comparison, my mom is a lot healthier than now. You almost have to enjoy the now because the next "now" is... it is what it is.... One would be doing a disservice to ourselves if we think that things are gonna get "better."*

Casey also talked about learning to "enjoy the now" with her partner, despite grappling with the loss of what he and their relationship used to be like:

> *We can still sit together on the couch in a dark room watching a TV show with subtitles and you're like, this is a nice quiet moment.... You always kind of glorify your next stage of life. And I'm like, "Well, I'm in it right now. I need to enjoy this right now. Because who knows what's going to happen next?"*

I asked Debbie, now that she is aware of the gradual loss she's been experiencing, how she has learned to cope:

> *Lots of love and support from other people in my life.... I think when the person that you care for—especially with a parent—if they can't really be in that role for you in some ways anymore, it's having to figure out how to still get those needs met for yourself, in the way that you care for yourself or in*

the supports in your life. It's a big thing that I've learned, is really needing to be able to ask for what I need from other people in my life so that I am feeling like emotional needs are getting met.... Sometimes just a really big hug and you're okay.

AMBIGUOUS LOSS OF YOUR OWN EXPECTATIONS... DREAMS...THE LIFE YOU THOUGHT YOU'D HAVE

"You're just miserable if you lose hope, right? If I just say, 'Oh, well, I guess I'm never having a cat.' That's such a dumb small thing, but it's almost like a grief, right? If you give up on these tiny little goals and these tiny, tiny wants?" Casey, who cares for her husband, is one of the most optimistic young women I've met, but in the face of it she grieves for a lot: not only her partner's "old" self, but hers as well. Her husband was not chronically ill through much of their relationship prior to our speaking. In our talks together, before their wedding, she told me about "the death of our dreams" in such a matter-of-fact way that, hearing it from a woman in her thirties who was about to embark on a new marriage, was jarring. She said it took her over a year to realize his condition might last forever. She'd always dreamt of having a wedding with everyone she loves, living in the country, having kids—all things she's realized his illness probably makes unfeasible. On top of that: she's always wanted a cat.

I love animals so much. I've always wanted a dog or a cat or multiples of both. And so since [my husband] got sick...his body is just so sensitive to everything. I went to go housesit for someone's cat and came back and touched a pillow and some of the cat hair got on the pillow and he just was miserable for the whole rest of the day. A cat is such a tiny goal and I want it so much, but it just physically is not possible right now. So you just kind of have to hold on to these seemingly little dreams that are big deals to you.

The family she thought she would have...the lost time with friends and the relationship she used to have with her partner...the cat. All these are instances of grief and another form of ambiguous loss. I often hear caregivers our age, when they are honest with themselves out loud, express grief for the life they thought they'd have. When you are still in the development stages of your life and those expectations get set aside— or dashed completely—for reasons that feel out of your control, there's a major sense of loss.

"Anytime we're forfeiting an ideal or a vision we have for ourselves, it's a mourning process," therapist Dr. Lisa said. "And there's resentment that comes up, and there's loss that comes up, and there's fear and there's anger. And I think that those are all normative places to land." In this generation used to manifesting, of creating visions boards, or just being humans with desires, the images we have in our minds of our hopes and dreams can be very powerful; realizing they are no longer feasible can be devastating.

"WHAT ABOUT A HAIRLESS CAT?" I OFFERED TO CASEY. I DIDN'T WANT her to give up hope either.

"Anything that helps you think more creatively and develop a really dark sense of humor," she said, laughing. Instead, she asks friends to send pictures of their animals to cheer her up.

One caregiving resource warned that giving these previous dreams a lot of time and energy keeps you rooted in the past and uses energy you need to cope in the present.[10] They advised striking a balance between grieving the loss of things you hoped for, or even planned, and living in the present moment; this allows you not to miss new and different opportunities available to you. Dr. Lisa mentioned, also, that you may be "mourning the possibility...of what could have been, not necessarily the guarantee that it would have."

My personal belief is that you don't need to discard those ideas or dreams entirely; just allow them to change shape in ways that you may not have prepared for but that are still feasible. Dr. Lisa referred to this as "finding the reframe." After mourning what will not be, "find a reframe of how to create meaningful moments instead, or in spite, of the fact that maybe [you] didn't get to date wildly in your twenties or... [you] won't be having children. But [you'll] still know how to give love and receive love, or whatever [your] reframe is that creates closure for what wasn't and provides meaning for what is and what will be."

Hope is a powerful resource when it comes to caregiving, and not losing hope—for the health of your family member, for yourself—is critical in coping. I noticed Kaci, caring for her mom since her twenties, had developed an optimism when readjusting her goals to fit her reality. Just because she did not do certain activities or take certain trips when she thought she would doesn't mean she'll never do them. She accepts that "my timeline may not look like everybody else's anymore."

I asked Kaci what she thinks about when she thinks about her future. She told me that it's difficult; not imagining what she wants but to think about a time post-caregiving:

This came up a few weeks ago with my boyfriend. He was like, "Well, you know, maybe someday we won't be living in Rochester. We're gonna be doing all these things." And I was like, "You have to realize having that conversation with me is really hard because what that means is my mom is not alive." And I think sometimes people don't understand that. I can have these dreams, but to actually say what it would take for me to have them [come true] is also extremely depressing.

ANTICIPATORY GRIEF

Erica lost her father to cancer years ago; after he passed, her mom was diagnosed with multiple system atrophy, for which there's no cure and no way of slowing its progression. Even though her mom needed round-the-clock care to continue living at home, Erica hoped her mother still had years of life ahead of her. Yet when Erica thought about her future wedding, she already imagined what it will be like if her mom is no longer alive. "I have a wonderful boyfriend that I live with and...I don't know, if my mom's not around, if I want to have a big wedding. Because [if] my dad's not here, my mom isn't here, [I think] that I just want to do something small."

This is anticipatory grief.

Anticipatory grief is when you grieve for someone who is still alive, and it's common among caregivers—particularly those of us with a loved one diagnosed with a terminal or degenerative illness.[11] When faced with an impending loss, your mind projects what life will be like "after." Signs of anticipatory grief can include extreme concern for the person you care for, frequent thoughts about the person's death and how you will adjust, and guilt or shame for "wishing it were over."[12] Your mind may begin to go there way before death is on the horizon; changes in the person's abilities or how they relate to you (as in ambiguous loss) can trigger thoughts of their death and your life after. Anticipatory grief is a completely normal emotion, but it's important to monitor how much of your thoughts it consumes: chronic anticipatory grief can lead to depression.[13]

One positive thing about anticipatory grief: it can allow us to adjust to the eventual loss of the person and say the things we want to before they are gone.[14] It's an opportunity to resolve past issues with them in a way that is not possible when a loss is sudden. But this doesn't take into account a person with cognitive decline; a resolution in the relationship is not available in the same way as before the disease. "There are certain things about relationships we can't really repair anymore, or actively work on, because the person's not able. Like they're not able to do it," Debbie said of her mom's dementia. It's a source of sadness for Debbie.

Christina Irving says that when confronted with feelings of anticipatory loss, connecting with other caregivers can be helpful; they may understand this grief that is often overlooked by society at large. "Allow yourself to grieve for what you've lost and what you know is coming; those losses are real and valid even if we don't have condolence cards that recognize it. But then, at the same time, find those moments of joy, contentment, or gratitude [with your loved one] where you can."

GRIEF IN BEREAVEMENT

One surprising thing I've observed while moderating Caregiver Collective is the number of people who join *after* being a caregiver. Often still processing the journey they have been on, they report feeling "lost" without caregiving. Coupled with the relief they may now experience, that their loved one's suffering is over, they feel the absence of what had consumed so much of their lives prior.

Not what you expected for a caregiver's grief in bereavement, is it? But this is an additional loss I've heard many times and, in ways, felt myself: the loss of the caregiver role. After devoting time, energy, emotion, and all mental resources, the need is suddenly…gone. The skills you acquired, the tips and tricks, no longer necessary. Not to mention, it was a role that bound you to a person you love. There is an intimacy acquired through caregiving that you may not share in the same way with anyone else.

Some people find it impossible to maintain their own identity outside of caregiving, so the shock of no longer being a caregiver can leave a particular void the person must now learn how to fill. Maybe you're forty and began caring at twenty-five…do you still like to do the same things as back then? What do you like to do now? Your friends have had kids in that time, so what is your relationship with them going to be like now? There are a multitude of ways grieving the caregiver role can look, questions that can arise.

Christina Irving says maintaining your own sense of identity while you are still caregiving and pursuing your own interests outside of your role as much as you can, even if the way you do so looks different from how you would before, can be helpful in this transition. "It's hard for caregivers to figure out what their life looks like now after what has often been years of caregiving," Irving said. "You may no longer be a caregiver, but what are the skills you've gained? What have you learned about yourself through the process? There's a reason why so many former caregivers choose to work in this space when their caregiving is done. Give yourself time to figure out what you want to do next, and part of that time may be reflecting on what's important to you now and how you want to spend your time and energy."

Grief after a person has passed is an entire bookstore aisle in itself, but from the perspective of caregivers our age, there are some things I believe it's important to touch on here. In general, grief in bereavement can present in many ways; you may experience some or all of the signs. Maybe you experience one display of grief one day, then the next you go through the full range. Here are some signs and symptoms of grief:[15]

Feeling emotionally numb
Being unable to believe the loss occurred: shock, disbelief, or denial
Anxiety from the distress of being separated from the loved one
Crying, sighing
Dreams, illusions, or even hallucinations of the deceased
Looking for places or things shared with the deceased
Mourning (showing grief in public) with feeling depressed
Feelings of acceptance

In general, studies have shown that younger bereaved people have more problems after a loss than older bereaved people do, such as severe health problems, grief symptoms, or other mental and physical symptoms.[16] Also, those who found benefits or positive aspects to being a caregiver (like a closer connection with the person they cared for or the time spent together) had higher levels of depression and grief in bereavement.[17] I share this with you to send up flares. For those of you providing care now, I don't intend to kick you into anticipatory grief, but I do encourage you to listen to Alex, who shared insight from her grief after her mother passed:

One of my regrets (but again, where do you find the time?)—I went to one or two grief groups and I kind of half-heartedly tried to find a therapist, but I never really had that emotional support team. It took me a long time to get that in place, which I now have a great therapist that I talk to about grief and I've tried energy workers and I'm into all the healers and all this stuff. But I kind of wish I had put some of that in place earlier.

Support doesn't need to look like energy healers (although I lived in Los Angeles for over a decade, so you know I also have my roster), but the message is: put support into place now, so it's already there when you need it. Finding a person or place to turn to when you are grieving can require energy that, on some days, you won't have. Friends and family of caregivers or those in bereavement: lend a guiding hand (not an overbearing one) to help them.

CHAPTER 16

WE'RE FEELING *PISSED OFF*

O NE CAREGIVER COLLECTIVE POST GAINED TRACTION SO FAST AND furiously, I logged in to see what everyone was commenting on. It was the share of a Medium essay on caregiving, specifically about people who encouraged the author to view caregiving as a "gift."[1] These well-meaning friends encouraged "silver linings." The notion was met with rage.

"These comments are always made with the best of intentions," the author, a caregiver in her early thirties, wrote. "But here is the truth: I don't feel blessed, I don't find comfort in how things could be worse, I often struggle to see how complex challenges will work out, and I can feel however I want to!"

The title of the essay is, fittingly, "Caregivers Are Over Your Toxic Positivity." Before this essay, the thousand-plus members of the Collective hadn't really acknowledged what they felt about being told to look on the bright side, so the group's quick reaction was a bit surprising. I asked the author of this essay, Debbie Malley (a group member herself), what led her to write it.

"I remember, I was just angry," she said.

And she wasn't the only one. Here are some of the responses to her essay:

This!!! I am no longer a caregiver as my dad died a year and a half ago (?! what is time), but I remember this feeling so well. It still makes my blood boil. "It'll get better," mfer, he has dementia, what are you talking about!

Every time somebody says "everything happens for a reason," I want to slap them.

Caregivers don't often admit in earshot of other people that we are pissed off. Not always, but regularly. And particularly, it seems, when we're on the receiving end of this unhelpful "positivity"...which caregivers our age are, regularly. Conversations that are dead-ended with a "Look on the bright side" or "It'll get better!"—we receive these flat notions of good faith not only from people with no care experience but also from older caregivers who assume our situation is not as tough as theirs. We're young, how could it be? Statements like "You're lucky, you don't know how bad it can be" come from caregivers who, unlike us, most often had time to develop their own lives before taking on the job themselves. The entire exchange can feel like someone's looking right at you but doesn't *see* you. Yet we know they (hopefully?) come from a good place, so it can be hard to be told something well-meaning and then admit the response in your head is *Fuck. Off.*

"It's like anger at not being seen and feeling like you're being truly heard, what's happening to you," Debbie said. That dissonance between the difficult experience you're living and someone's perception of it seemed to be at the root of a lot of anger and resentment for the caregivers I've spoken with. So if it regularly enrages those of us caring, why don't we speak up? Debbie weighed in:

It's a difficult conversation to have, even when it's a need of yours, to tell someone "the way you've been responding to me makes me feel worse." You know, that's not an easy thing to say.

Debbie believes the people in her life are concerned and trying to understand but fall short in their attempts. She attributed some of this to our age and a life experience out of whack with those around her:

Most of my peers have not been through this type of experience, and I think that's where some of those sort of toxic positivity platitudes come in. Because people don't know what else to say sometimes. And I think there's good intention there, but it can feel really invalidating.

It's understandable if someone in your life doesn't know what to say; these things are difficult and, in turn, difficult to put words to. Casey, who cares for her chronically ill husband, thinks her own rosy demeanor has increased the misunderstanding friends have of the couple's reality. She and her husband don't share many of the details of his illness or of her caregiving with their social circle; instead, they often lean into portraying more upbeat representations of themselves. She believes that if she admitted to friends and family that this has been the "worst two years of [her] life," they wouldn't know how to process that uncomfortable truth.

THAT'S A THING ABOUT TOXIC POSITIVITY, IT'S A DOUBLE-EDGED SWORD: caregivers engage in it, too. On the caregiver end, there's often an instinct that when somebody asks you how you are, you say "good" and paint over the reality. It's a missed opportunity to be honest, but it can be motivated by a variety of reasons that feel, in that moment, more worthwhile: You don't want to talk about it then. You're not comfortable sharing specific details or with the person asking. You don't have the energy. You wish, just for a moment, not to think about it.

Anger, it seems, is often rooted in a disconnect of understanding what the person doing the care work is *actually* doing, the emotional (and physical) heft of the experience they undergo. This disconnect can exist between the caregiver and coworkers, friends, even family and can cause strain along the way when the caregiver's building resentment explodes. Brandon experienced this with his brothers.

One thing I've observed about Brandon over the years of knowing him through caregiving, he's great at making lemonade. When Brandon first shared the journey he took uprooting his life in New York to move back in with his mom in Michigan, the tone he took was really... well, bright-eyed. He told me that, at the time, he saw caring for his mom as an opportunity to have time to write the book he'd always wanted to write and to reconnect with friends from high school who still lived in the area. Living in Michigan again, or with his mom, wasn't in his plans, but it wasn't so bad. He sounded like a problem solver who looked for opportunity in where life led him.

The next time we spoke was different. The same story, though this time through a lens of how his two brothers maintained their own lives while his was turned upside down. With this retelling, Brandon was furious:

> *In the fight that I had with my brother I would just be so angry. I'd be angry that he didn't "get it" more. Because I would downplay how hard things were. I didn't want him to feel bad, you know, so I would downplay that, like, "No, I never wanted to fucking move away from New York." I lived there [Michigan] a decade prior, you know, great place to visit. See my old friends. I don't want to live there. . . . I would downplay things now by saying, "Oh, I have more time to do my writing." I would just be surprised that even with the people that were close to me, sometimes they wouldn't see the true sacrifice being made, you know. Even if I was downplaying it for my own sake.*

As Brandon retold his story without the rosy lens, he grew more incensed. How could his brother not understand the gravity of the changes Brandon was making to his own life, right in front of him? How could he not take a moment to consider what Brandon was going through to help their mom? I found it interesting that Brandon didn't tell his brother the reality of how he felt; instead, he painted this picture so that his brother wouldn't "feel bad" but then assumed he'd get it. And when his brother didn't, Brandon was furious. There's that disconnect. That it was fostered by Brandon's own share to his brother isn't surprising—any caregiver I know has at one time or another glossed over their reality for, what they think, is the benefit of the listener. Or because they don't want to sound like they're complaining. It goes against what is at the heart of what the caregiver *actually wants*.

In my experience, the rosy outlook is not always a lie of convenience but a hope for how you would like it to be; it's leaning into what is, on some days, true. But the feelings of anger and resentment are also real. The conflicting emotions live alongside each other, the disconnect also internal. Both versions of Brandon's story felt honest.

ROOT OF ANGER: UNSEEN AND UNHEARD

Primarily, caregiving adults in their twenties, thirties, and early forties often feel like their personal compromises aren't acknowledged. They're not looking for medals; they just want to feel heard when they say, "This is hard," or, "I'm thirty and feel like I'm eighty," or whichever uncomfortable truth they want to get off their chest. People want to express what they are going through and hear an honest response. (Or, like Brandon, even when they don't explicitly state it, they hope you'll take an objective look at their situation.) Megan, who cared for her mom who had Parkinson's, said, "I find it really compelling how noncaregiver's toxic positivity is just unbearable, but [a] fellow caregiver's brutal honesty/negativity ('Trust me, it gets so much worse') can make you feel so much better?! I guess it shows the healing powers of empathy and feeling understood and 'seen.'" Just like when you were a teenager, feeling unheard can quickly escalate to anger and frustration—especially when that lack of acknowledgment becomes routine.

"I harbored a lot of resentment, I would say, for my situation," Kaci told me, "sometimes where I felt like I'd given up a lot of my life and I don't always feel appreciated." Kaci has forgone a lot for her mother's care; she's done what she feels needed to be done but would just like the toll it's taken on her to be acknowledged. Instead, she gets the sense it's expected of her: her mother cared for her grandparents in their old age, so now it was Kaci's turn. In their Polish background, culturally that was the way.

"I think to her," Kaci said of her mother, "it was almost like a 'this is expected of you' kind of situation, because that was a lot of it where she

was like, 'Well, I did this for Gram and Dido' [Kaci's grandparents]....
And then I finally snapped and was like, 'Yeah, Mom, you did it for one
year. This has been eleven years of my life, that's what you don't understand.' She did it for one year." Because Kaci began caring for her mom
in her twenties and her mom's longevity, thankfully, seems pretty good,
Kaci will most likely be caregiving for decades. That is a long time for the
financial, relational, and physical tensions to build, for anger and resentment to accumulate, and a lot of youth sacrificed in exchange for a steep
learning curve. "She was in her fifties, I was in my twenties, and I think
sometimes people forget the age piece because I remember somebody
at work was like, 'Well, I did that with my mom.' And I'm like, you're
sixty-seven. You did it with your mom last year." Again, there's that piece
of not feeling seen.

Kaci also notices this when people in her life make casual comments
that, as Debbie mentioned, invalidate Kaci's experience:

> I just remember my ex's cousin had kids, I think their kids were, like, five
> or six or a little bit older. I remember being at a family event and I was like,
> "Oh gosh, I get home so tired" and she's like, "You don't even know what
> tired is. Wait till you have children." And that really got to me because peo-
> ple say that to me all the time.

OTHER CAUSES OF ANGER

At the end of our ropes. Overlooked and underappreciated. This pushes a
lot of us over the edge, but there are other causes of anger, too: my anger
was often born out of frustration for what I had no control over, and I
lashed out. I hear a lot of anger from young adults who feel taken advantage of—not by the person they care for, but by the other family members
who do little or nothing at all to help. Some caregivers voice anger for the
family members who ask when they'll finally start a family of their own.
How could they possibly afford the time, money, or energy when they're

caregiving all the time, and without help from the person inquiring? How can they be expected to fulfill all their expectations? It's anger at them for expecting and not helping, and it's anger in general over what a caregiver feels they are missing out on.

Although Michelle and her dad were the caregivers to her mom, Michelle knew her mom could help at home, even if just in small ways. Michelle expressed resentment that her mother wouldn't pitch in and instead put everything on Michelle and her dad to handle. Casey expressed anger and frustration at media depictions of illness: "I'm not super into Hallmark movies, but they almost play illness or hospitalizations...lightly, as this problem to overcome." She feels illness is treated as a gimmick instead of life altering.

I also felt angry when I thought about my career. I had already been frustrated in my job and, in comparison to illness and family, it seemed like bullshit. Some things at work were regarded as so important, but in the grand scheme of life were so meaningless, and I was angry other people couldn't see that. I'd have thoughts like, *How could you complain about this insignificant thing and how it feels like the end of the world when it means nothing to me? And shouldn't this trivial thing also mean little to you?* Heavy medical realities and fears were at the top of my priority list and consciousness at the time; I didn't have room or patience for life's everyday concerns.

I remember, somewhere around this time (whether my dad had passed away yet or not I'm not sure) a friend said to me, thoughtfully: "You're so *angry*." I had no idea what she was talking about. I felt misjudged. I know that, in the core of my being, I am not an angry person. I was just *sad*. Some days it exploded in tears, some days the tears just welled and were quickly swiped away with the back of my hand, and some days there were fists punched against thighs or sofa cushions. Angry wasn't what I was; anger was just a way it was expressed. Sometimes we reach for the easy emotion because to acknowledge the real one hurts too badly.

Christina Irving, of Family Caregiver Alliance, says if others notice a new frequency or intensity in our anger or resentment, or we notice it within ourselves, or if we're angering easily, to take that as a warning sign:

What can be helpful for caregivers is being able to recognize their emotions, their well-being, early on.... It makes it easier for people to notice when those emotional reactions start to increase. When people kind of hold on to it, you're more likely to have those eruptions of the emotions. And it also means that people aren't going to notice in themselves that they're feeling more and more frustration, anger, resentment, grief, guilt, all that because they haven't noticed what [their] baseline was for that. So finding those ways to kind of check in about, "Okay, how am I doing? I noticed that I'm more emotional than I used to be, that's new." And again, taking that as a message there's something going on. "Do I need to talk to somebody? Do I need to find ways to get more breaks? Do I need to find outlets, some of those more wellness activities that I need to build into my life in some way, shape, or form? Because this is not normal for me, this is different." So just being able to notice and know what's my baseline and what has started to change.

She recommends that if you are noticing a new frequency or intensity of your anger, then it's time to bring in outside help and support, like a therapist, to help you process your emotions and navigate how to move forward. If you don't address these emotions, they may affect your health or lead to burnout.

I asked Debbie Malley what the result of sharing her Medium article with people in her life was. Did it help at all? Did they follow through, or was it met with more misalignment? Here's what she said:

It has led to some better understanding and some really nice moments of connection. If I think about some people that I've talked to, it takes it beyond the surface level conversation which I've really appreciated. So I think there has been some positive response, like that I feel more connected to that person after talking more authentically. It's not a conversation I've had with everybody. I saw [with] many friends, family members in my life that we just haven't really gotten there. Which I'm okay with ... I don't need that level of being seen, supported by everybody. I think if I just have a couple of people in my corner who are willing to [be], that's enough for me.

PART FOUR

ARE CAREER AND FINANCIAL GOALS A MYTH FOR US?

CHAPTER 17

CARE VERSUS CAREER (OR, THE CAREER COMPROMISE)

H ERE'S A BLUNT TRUTH: CAREGIVING CAN ROB US OF CAREER OR CON-
tinuing education goals early on. Throughout my time meeting people of my generation who provide family care, I've been stunned to see
how many careers were put on hold, shuttled aside, or grieved as unat-
tainable. I spoke with a young woman forced to drop out of graduate
school because missing class to provide emergency family care wasn't
recognized as a valid excuse by her professor or the administration; she
was flunked for attendance but couldn't financially afford to repeat the
class. Ultimately, she sacrificed the credits she'd earned and dropped
out entirely.

I don't know how many people I've met who told me they had put
the pieces in place to pursue their dreams, but an emergency phone call
changed everything. Plans are dropped or shoved aside for the immediate need of tending to someone's health; for some, indefinitely. Career
paths are interrupted and the fallout doesn't just hit our hearts but also
threatens our bank accounts and health insurance. When you examine
the situation, care and career are at odds...usually with one winning out
over the other. It's mind-boggling that this is an ultimatum so many people in their *twenties and thirties* are confronting, before they've had the
opportunity to explore and build work experience or financial stability,

particularly when employment stability is not something our generation has enjoyed much of.

In 2016, the *Detroit Free Press* published an article entitled "Millenials Aim to Attain American Dream, but Can They?"[1] It stated, "Millennials—perhaps more than any other generation—grew up being told: If you can dream it, you can achieve it." My generation was sold on advanced education to get you there. For some eighties and nineties kids, the dream came true: I was at the University of Michigan when Facebook was started by another college student at another school, I had graduated when it took off. Throughout American history, we have examples of hard workers with a clever idea who bootstrapped their way to success.

For others, when we graduated from college or entered the workforce after high school, ready to take on the world, there were few jobs. For years. The eldest of us emerged into the workforce during the post-9/11 recession and were warned to expect lower starting wages; then the Great Recession hit in 2007, striking another major blow to jobseekers. The youngest of us had been working for only a few years max when COVID turned the working world upside down.

Our bad timing alone has major implications: entering the labor force during a recession can affect your entire career. Across race and education levels, those entering the labor market during a recession have had much weaker earnings and career advancement—not just initially, but over the long term.[2] For those who graduated from college, initial earnings losses are significant (about 9 percent annually), and the reduction in hourly wages or annual incomes can last into their mid-forties.[3] Someone in this position tries to catch up by switching companies more frequently than someone who graduates in better economic times. Basically, taking the job you can get, one that is not as well-paying as it would've been under better economic circumstances, is the launchpad for the rest of your career and impacts your career trajectory, quality of future opportunities, and income. Oh, and savings and benefits. And that's all just because of the year you graduated college or were ready to begin your life of employment.

This jobs landscape shaped the relationship Millennials have with work and employers. It explains the attitudes we approach our careers with—and explains the reasoning behind the negative stereotypes that call us disloyal, fly-by-night employees and the "job-hopping generation."[4] Research by Boston College sheds some light:

> Beginning in the late 20th century, a dramatic shift occurred in the relationship between careers and employers as significant organizational downsizing reached record levels in the 1990s and early 2000s.... As a result of these changes, employees realized that the employment contract—the belief that good employees would be rewarded with job security—was dramatically altered, and may have resulted in young professionals seeing themselves more as free agents, willing to change jobs frequently to reach their career goals.[5]

Ah-*ha*. Millennials, it seems, have not been offered what previous generations took for granted: job security. Low expectations of company security or loyalty can explain why Millennials predominantly want two things from their careers: flexibility and work-life balance—and, in the context of our post-COVID record-inflation economy, I'd bet *living wage* is also high on that list. Currently, we are in the years of our life that have the capacity to be our most productive and highest earning but are racked by record inflation. How to pay for groceries is a nightly topic on the news; many of us haven't built up savings to dip into. Lower rents in the immediate COVID aftermath (if you got one) have shot back up, groceries no matter where you shop are a zillion dollars. Getting through today is expensive; saving for tomorrow is something we'll have to deal with... tomorrow.

Given this economic instability, a Millennial worker can feel desperate for financial control. You can understand, then, the allure of striking out as an entrepreneur to be your own boss or the need to enter the gig economy. You can also understand how, for someone early in their career and employment life, all of this is stressful even before family care is added into the mix.

CAREGIVING AND OUR CAREER AT ODDS

With millions of us in this position, it's crucial we understand how our careers impact our care—and how our care impacts our careers. Even before COVID, the situation of balancing care with career for young (or younger) adults was not good. On average, in addition to full-time jobs, Millennials provided enough hours of unpaid care per week (approximately 21 hours) for it to be considered a part-time job.

Chelsea was in her early twenties and working her first full-time job at a law firm when her dad had a massive stroke. He was hospitalized for weeks and she took time off to care for him. When she returned to the office, things became even more stressful: her boss was clear that if she kept leaving the office to care for her dad, she would lose her job. Chelsea was overwhelmed by the information, it didn't feel real. She found it difficult to concentrate, often breaking into tears.

Chelsea didn't have access to paid or unpaid leave for family medical care, she was at the mercy of her boss's discretion and, it was made clear, under threat of termination if she continued to tend to her dad. (To those of you who are versed in caregiver workplace protections and are wondering: *But what about FMLA?*, we're getting into that in a minute.)

She's far from alone: Millennials are more likely than other generations to balance caregiving with employment *but also* more likely to receive negative workplace consequences as a result.[6] According to AARP, these negative repercussions take the form of warnings about performance or attendance, denied promotions, being fired, or stopping work entirely. Any of these can impact income, career progression, and growth and could jeopardize long-term financial security. Remember, a lot of these Millennials entered the workforce during a recession and already experienced a stunted start; for all of them, care is expensive.

In 2018, one in three Millennial caregivers earned less than $30,000 a year.[7] It's hard to imagine any of them could afford a gut punch to their income and savings or to lose their job. Seventy percent of a person's overall wage growth occurs in their first ten years of employment; interruptions during that time can be costly.[8] On top of it, a lot of people tie personal value and identity to their careers or degrees, especially in American society. Consistently being held down or held back can negatively affect your feelings of self-worth. It deepens the chasm between those who provide care and those who don't, both fiscally and emotionally.

What are employers warning these employed Millennials about? Off the bat: arriving late, leaving early, or cutting back on work hours. And these grievances are accurate: more than half of employed Millennial caregivers reported doing at least one of these. It's reasonable: doctor appointments can only be scheduled during work hours, medical emergencies happen when they happen and can interrupt the workday; if there's a major medical incident in your family, like Chelsea, you may be out of the office for days, at least.

When her dad had the stroke, Chelsea was young—and young in her career—and didn't have much experience. It can be assumed that it would be easier for her boss to replace her than if she were a more seasoned employee. This is why, I believe, Millennials have faced higher workplace repercussions as a result of care: because our age and experience, at least for those of us younger, make us seem more expendable. Another reason is our silence at work about caregiving: Afraid of being stigmatized as not wholly committed to their job, most often Millennials don't share what's going on at home and push through silently at the office. They are less likely to share at work that they are a family caregiver than Boomers are; in fact, unlike Chelsea, less than half of Millennial caregivers had told their work supervisor.[9] When they show up late or leave early or miss days, their bosses often don't know *why*.

Many don't even discuss caregiving with coworkers. Michelle said she didn't for a long time despite when caring for her mom took her away from the office and affected her work life. She didn't think it would be accepted as "workplace appropriate."

"All my caregiving is like a second job, it's like another side of me essentially, and I think something that stood out to me in the workplace [is] there's a real openness to sharing about, 'Man, my kid was crying all night.' Sharing that, and that being okay. But I feel like on the flip side of it, from a caregiving perspective... it's not as readily acceptable to share like, 'Yeah, I was up all night helping [my mom] with her treatment.'" Though both childcare and eldercare are family care, one seemed to be acceptable office chitchat and the other was not.

Balancing the two worlds can be untenable; it can result in feeling sick or exhausted at work, not operating at 100 percent. Something has to give somewhere. Some of us couldn't manage full-time jobs with care so cut back employment hours, which can disqualify us from our health insurance and put our now lower income below the national median. Other times, the cost of paid care becomes a consideration that outweighs career aspirations: if the salary coming in doesn't offset the cost for care going out, it can be an economic decision to stay home. Pre-COVID, half of caregivers ages twenty-six to thirty-five had already left a job because of caregiving, with women and people of color being disproportionately affected.[10] Another (surprising?) group: highly paid young men. One study by Harvard found that, prepandemic, a significant number of highly paid men between the ages of twenty-five and thirty-five had left a job for caregiving, though reports show women bear the brunt of caregiving in the total population.[11]

THE BOTTOM LINE: EVEN IN DECENT ECONOMIC TIMES, WHEN YOU TAKE on family care at our age it often translates into job and income insecurity.

THE WORK CRISIS THAT IMPACTED OUR CARE

You might assume that the halt of business during COVID, followed by the temporary transition to work-from-home (for those nonessential workers), eased the balancing act for employed individuals who were also providing family care work…and for some it did, but for most: au contraire. At a time when young adults were most affected by pandemic-related job loss, caregiving duties intensified.[12] Previous support, like paid aides or a neighbor who helped out, was no longer safely available; some families chose to move loved ones out of living facilities and in with them. For those living or indefinitely staying with the person they were caring for, care became 24/7. The family caregivers who cared for someone outside of their home needed to figure out how to keep that person safe and cared for remotely, a set of conditions new to everyone, and terrifying. Those who retained employment or kept hustling to keep their self-owned business from collapsing became chronically overwhelmed (polite word) by the overlap of "jobs."

One bright spot was that work-from-home became possible. Employed people who needed to provide family care had been requesting this consideration *for years*—they did not want to stop working, but before the pandemic, there were times they absolutely needed to be at home or at a hospital bedside and needed that flexibility. For a Millennial, this was not a crazy ask: pre-COVID, Millennials in the workforce were trending toward a remote work environment, while older managers were resistant and often told them no. What "wasn't possible" for caregivers before the pandemic became quickly routine for everyone once lockdowns began.

Anyone whose employment could only operate outside of the home, like an essential worker's, had to weigh paycheck against safety when the threat of leaving the home was too great for high-risk family members. I remember one young business owner couldn't visit the store she owned, where she was needed, and each day tried to evaluate when it would be safe enough to return to keep the lights on.

Still, many caregivers tried to stay optimistic. At the height of the lockdowns, I spoke with John. Thirty-seven at the time, he cared for both parents who had each had a stroke within a month of each other. Before they required care, John had a job in politics and was enrolled in a graduate program in his home state of New Jersey; he left both to provide full-time care in their home, not wanting to put them in a nursing home. Continuing his care into lockdowns presented a new set of difficulties to keeping the family safe, and now without the help of aides and extended family he had come to count on. It had been a long road for John; then, tragically, his father died, and then his mother, while we were still in the midst of the pandemic. For the first time in years, John was available to reenter the workforce—and some essential services were hiring.

"I have learned not to let adversity deter me," he said. "Family caregivers make enough sacrifices regarding work schedules and cannot afford to be passive about our future opportunities because of this crisis." John took a job at an Amazon distribution center, one of the few places in need of workers at the time, and he looked forward to getting back out there.

THAT "WEIRD STIGMA" YOU FACE IS WORKPLACE BIAS

Once the pandemic's first wave quelled, some employers no longer allowed remote work, but caregivers didn't yet feel it was safe enough to return to the office or classroom, so their jobs were, again, in the crosshairs. Casey was allowed to continue working from home, but the concession came with repercussions—and illuminated how much care had already impacted her career.

Casey is thirty-five, which means she entered the workforce around 2010, squarely in the aftermath of the Great Recession. When her husband (then-boyfriend) first fell chronically ill and she moved in to care for him, she worked for a small web design company where she had already been employed for nine years. She said that it was a "really great first job" but that her salary and benefits hadn't kept up with her performance growth. The company didn't offer health benefits or a 401(k); all her medical expenses, including any medical emergencies, she paid for out of pocket. Casey's boss knew she was caregiving for her boyfriend. When workers returned to the office after lockdowns, Casey requested to stay remote. It was the only way to continue providing the care her boyfriend needed, often doctor visits popped up last minute and they were urgent.

She began to notice she was treated differently from those who returned to the office, but she felt stuck:

> Occasionally, I'll talk to my other coworkers, and we'll talk about raises or extra benefits that they're getting. And the only difference I can see is that I'm the only one working remote and caregiving. And I've heard other coworkers say that my boss doesn't quite know what to do with me because he's giving me the benefit of working from home. But we get so little vacation, that most of the time when I take my boyfriend to appointments, I'm not being paid for that time and so it is a financial burden as well.

She considered going back to the office but thought, with her boyfriend's care and compromised immunity, it would be too draining. Even fully remote, Casey had a hard time balancing the two roles; she thinks that working for a smaller business was the reason they didn't have any accommodations in place for someone in her position.

"I'm taking a lot of unpaid leave. And it just felt like there was this weird stigma around me at the office, that I was somehow getting special treatment for getting to work [from] home even though I was basically working two jobs, right? . . . It just felt like there wasn't a lot of support there." That "stigma" she faced is called workplace bias. Being passed over for project opportunities and overlooked for raises received by coworkers who had worked there for a shorter period—these are examples of workplace discrimination.

Depending on which state or city you live in, these acts may be frowned upon by your company's Human Resources department but be completely legal. The Americans with Disabilities Act (ADA) protects immediate relatives and spouses caring for someone with a disability; but Casey was not her boyfriend's spouse at the time, and because doctors have yet to officially diagnose his chronic illness, his disability paperwork had been held up. The Equal Employment Opportunity Commission (EEOC) would also not protect her. Let's say Casey's boss had thought that, because she's a woman in her thirties, she'll probably get pregnant soonish, and so he passes her over for a promotion. Under EEOC, that's against the law because an employer can't discriminate on the grounds of gender (or race or a slew of other identifiers). But if your boss learns that you are a caregiver and implicitly harbors unconscious (or, hell, conscious) bias that you will be less available for work and so withholds a promotion or job offer on those grounds? Legal, because the prejudice is based on *role*. Caregivers face this discrimination, particularly younger ones—especially because many employers have not wrapped their minds around the idea of a younger person being a caregiver.

Despite all this, Casey was afraid to leave that job. A job search is exhausting and would require even more energy of her. She also dealt with imposter syndrome because she didn't feel as qualified as she used to—without free time to advance her skills, she felt she'd grown stagnant and fallen behind. But it was a conversation with a former colleague that pushed Casey over the edge and into the job pool:

"I was talking with some of my other coworkers who had recently left the company and realizing how much less I was making and how many fewer benefits I had. They were making 30 percent more than I was, and they still didn't think it was enough for themselves. And I was like, 'Oh wow. Well, if that's not enough for them, then maybe I can do a little bit better.'" She began applying for fully remote jobs and did not tell potential employers that she was a caregiver.

WHY EMPLOYERS CAN GET AWAY WITH IT

I am not blind to the perspective of employers and supervisors: if you hire someone to fulfill a job responsibility and that person regularly arrives late and doesn't show the energy you expected, and that other employees have, you'd look at the bottom line and might consider replacing them. Let's put aside emotion and not jump to the conclusion that employers and supervisors are heartless. Let's even put aside that providing job flexibility to employees helps retain talent and actually benefits the company's bottom line and the economy (we'll get more into this later). But let's do consider that young adults providing care often feel like they don't have a choice: they've landed in caregiving situations they didn't seek out. No one chooses for their family member to be sick. No one wished for fewer care options. When the healthcare system makes our care role necessary for someone else's survival, how can companies be allowed to penalize us—particularly if, like Casey, we are still getting the job done well? Why is our ability to work (or earn a degree) resting on the attitudes of our company's (or university's) higher-ups, who can discriminate without repercussion before even considering concessions? How did our careers and our paychecks become so vulnerable, so expendable to others?

Because caregivers are not protected, not comprehensively, anyway. We already touched on how Chelsea's employer threatened her job, unethically, you could argue, but legally. She is one example of how business models in our nation can engage in discrimination without recourse, and the laws that enable them. In 2020, Senator Cory Booker introduced the Protecting Family Caregivers from Discrimination Act, which would (as its name sells) prohibit discrimination against employees for their caregiving responsibilities, prohibit employer retaliation if an employee seeks to enforce their rights, and establish a grant program to aid in combating employer discrimination.[13] The bill was reintroduced in 2022 but has yet to pass.

Some companies, including major corporations, do offer their employees benefits to help accommodate family care, such as more flexible hours and remote work. However, a (pre-COVID) Harvard study found that what was offered was often not enough; there was a "misalignment" between benefits employers thought their employees wanted and what the employees said would actually benefit them.[14] We are now in the employment aftermath of the pandemic, more aware of caregiving and more suited to understanding, and practicing, how to make flexibility in the workplace work. Yet, more employers are demanding a full back-to-the-office work culture, and the transition back has lasted longer than, probably, a lot of people first expected. It's too soon to tell whether the knowledge acquired during the pandemic will organically assist care-givers in the long run and flexible work policies will remain in place for them, even just as needed.

Inconsistent paid-leave policies are also to blame. As already mentioned, some families just cannot afford to take unpaid leave; the lack of income destabilizes their ability to pay utility bills or continue living in their home. Some workers are covered by the Family and Medical Leave Act (FMLA), a federal worker protection law that entitles eligible employees to job-protected leave in order to provide care for a family member and includes the continuation of health benefits.[15] FMLA offers twelve workweeks of leave in a twelve-month period for a spouse, child, or parent (including someone who filled the role of parent for you when you were a child, even if the relationship isn't biological or legal) and twenty-six workweeks for military caregivers. It prohibits demotion when you return to work. For some employees, it's a life preserver...but there's a catch: the leave is unpaid. Unless your employer provides paid care leave to use in tandem, you need to be able to "afford" the time away. Also, both you and your employer must be eligible. Private-sector employers must have at least fifty employees within a particular geographic radius (public agencies and local educational agencies are exempt from this minimum); employees must also fulfill requirements for eligibility, including working for that employer for at least twelve months beforehand. (Chelsea, for example, was not covered because the law firm that employed her had fewer than fifty employees.)

A comprehensive *paid family leave* policy that includes caregiving, regardless of who employs you, should be a *right* granted to all Americans but, at the moment, is a *benefit* only available state by state. The United States is the only country in the "developed" world not to offer any sort of national paid family leave program (while most of the thirty-eight Organisation for Economic Co-operation and Development [OECD] countries include caregiving, a select few cover only maternity or parental leave); we are only one of six in the world.[16] That's of all the countries on our planet. Taken in total, lack of support and protections for caregivers, whether employed or jobseekers, creates this care-or-career conundrum that—as we've seen—disproportionately affects our generation.

HOW SOME OF US MAKE IT WORK

Lizzie Prioritized a Job with Work-Life Balance Before Care Was in the Picture

It was weighing family care against career that made Lizzie a caregiver in the first place. After the lockdowns, when in-office work resumed for Lizzie and her husband, the couple had to consider childcare for their two small children. Vaccines were available for adults, but not yet for kids. Health safety was something they really considered: going back to the office meant putting the kids in day care unvaccinated.

"It was just a frustration of…a lot of decisions, whether the kids go to day care, or to stop working," she said. "We chose a day care and knew that there is an inherent risk in that." It was at day care that their youngest child contracted COVID; the child recovered, but the virus spread to Lizzie's husband, whose case developed into long COVID. Now his career is affected for the foreseeable future. Though it's been difficult, Lizzie has managed to keep her professional life on track thanks to an 80 percent workload schedule, a lifestyle change she had put into place before the pandemic and which she calls "a lifesaver."

Before she was caregiving, she said, "I was already feeling like, 'I work too much. I miss time with my kids. I don't want this to be my life.…I just want to slow down, but I would like to still have a career track.'… But I didn't want to take the pay cut. I still work 100 percent, I just do it at different times." Instead of switching to part-time, she decided to request going down to 80 percent but knew that if she asked her boss outright she'd most likely be denied. She decided to look for a counteroffer elsewhere to use as leverage in negotiating with her employer. Another company gave Lizzie the counteroffer with, to her surprise, a "pretty good pitch" to work for them. She accepted. At the time she didn't realize the job switch would be a lifeline. "Here I came in with about 80 percent [and] actually got a raise to go to 80 percent." She said her new coworkers are great. "They're totally supportive and they all know what's up because I've told them because I want them to know."

Even so, her thoughts have drifted to whether they secretly hold it against her. Regardless, she knows what good timing it was to already have a job that accommodated a work-life balance before care became necessary. Lizzie is a real-life example of how Millennials, caregiving or not, strive to balance work with home life, and how beneficial it can be (to the worker, to the business, to the labor economy) when it's attained.

Michelle Took FMLA Leave

When Michelle learned that her mother's renal disease had progressed to stage five and that her care needs were about to intensify, "I had a lot of momentum in my career," she said. "I had this trajectory, not only for the relocation [to Singapore], but just in terms of advancement. [But] you can't be considered for a promotion if you're taking, like, three days off, even if it is for family medical stuff. You're just not going to be able to be looked at [in] the same way your peers are who are fully present and full-time." Michelle is a self-proclaimed workaholic who, you'll remember, threw herself even more into her job to give herself a breath away from her care responsibilities and role. But her mom's needs, and both parents' dependence on Michelle, had ramped up so much it became impossible for her to do both. The frequency of doctor appointments increased drastically, and Michelle had little time even to sleep. "It was constantly taking off early or having late arrivals to work. But then when I got to work, I had trouble shifting gears and focusing and that led to later nights at work.... It was just this unending cycle where I was trying to keep up. When you're physically exhausted, you're mentally exhausted, and it was just a really bad recipe for disaster."

She knew she needed to make a change, even temporarily, to have enough time in the day (and night) for her mom's care without sacrificing her job. She made the decision to take leave under FMLA. For Michelle, it was a necessary stopgap solution to temporarily pause her job.

Since making that decision to take FMLA leave in 2019, Michelle observed that she needed to place better boundaries on how much care she was willing to take on herself; she needed to become better about telling her parents her limitations and asking for help. She doesn't think it was necessarily fair how much her family placed on her alone; expressing this is something she says she's working on. When I asked her, knowing what she knows now, what she would have done differently to protect herself from that work-care overload and burnout, she knew immediately: "FMLA much earlier. And not trying to deny that this situation was happening and real changes, real adjustments needed to be made in order to adapt with that new role that they were all taking on."

Jesus Pursued a Dream That Allowed Him to Be Available for Care

Jesus is a stand-up comic. He was in middle school when he began to help his mother manage her diabetes, doling out pills and, because his parents are native Spanish speakers, translating at doctor appointments. Later she developed a brain tumor; a somewhat unsuccessful surgery to remove it led to a host of other accelerating health issues, including Parkinson's. Later, his father was diagnosed with colon cancer. Jesus said he chose which college to attend based on being present to help with care; when he graduated he took an office job related to his degree but noticed care needs interfered. Taking responsibility for his parents' needs played a role in his decision of whether to pursue his stand-up dream full-time:

The caregiver situation almost lent [sic] itself for me to be a stand-up because I was taking a lot of time off of this super entry-level position that I was working in this marketing company...but I'm still doing open mics at the time. So I think one opportunity led to another and I just understood that stand-up was maybe my, I don't know, my ticket to taking care of my parents but also being able to live my dream.

Pursuing stand-up would leave his days free for care but would put pressure on him to make money with comedy at night. At first, it was a financial struggle. Jesus looks back on earlier times in his career, remembering what certain gigs did or didn't pay, and wonders how he managed to keep the lights on. Over time his career took off and he became more financially stable.

On top of the financial pressure, pursuing a career in comedy was a grind. His days were long and nights late. Being on the road meant someone would have to take over at home while he was gone. He began to think a nine-to-five without travel might be better, but then remembered that the schedule he had allowed him more days during the week to be at home. However, now if an emergency pops up when he's scheduled to perform, the show still goes on—with or without him. The audience is already in seats, and it's a huge pressure.

> *I can't tell you how many times I'm like minutes, moments, away from going onstage at a local comedy club here in LA and I'm getting a call. It's like "Hey, what's going on?" and I'm rattling off instructions. "Grab his pill crusher, put that in and grab the applesauce, give it to him. I'll call you right back. I gotta go onstage." That situation has happened…I don't know how many times.…And you go, you perform and it's like, you get a smile. There's a roomful of people laughing and smiling and having a great time and then you get off [stage] and then you walk to your car.…It's like, the switch as an artist is flipped aggressively up and down, on and off. You just have to hope that you have a good sturdy switch.*

He's now able to afford a separate home for his parents, whatever they need, and has hired home aides to relieve his day-to-day care responsibilities and allow more time for himself and his career. But even no longer living with his parents and having hired help, he realizes how intense caregiving still is. "We're caregivers through and through. I feel like there is no distinction…even at a distance the responsibilities, the weight of it all is the same."

If you're struggling to figure out how to balance it all, it can be inspiring just to hear there are others around your age in a similar situation who have figured out how to do it. Even still, you want to know *how*. For Jesus, it's a combination of organization and a mindset shift:

> *Between Google Calendar and an actual written calendar, you lay it all out and just hope that you're able to take care of all of it. It's never going to be perfect. And that's something that you're just going to have to come to terms with [as a caregiver]. Sometimes you're spending a little extra on plane tickets because you've got to come back at a certain time for this appointment and the ROI [return on investment] spending more money is peace of mind for yourself and the person you're caregiving, that you were there for that doctor's appointment, to be able to talk to him. But it's tough. Logistically, you just do your best.*

INCORPORATING CAREGIVING INTO CAREERS

Jesus's documentary about caregiving and his career, *Care to Laugh*, has led him to advocacy work around caregiving. He's not the only caregiver in our generation to incorporate their caregiving experience into their work.

With caregiving a bit more in the societal spotlight than it used to be, caregivers are emerging from the shadows and listing caregiving on their résumés, not only to explain a gap in employment but to promote management skills acquired at home. (As one job-seeking caregiver shared, employers should *want* to hire caregivers because they know how to manage time effectively and are accustomed to decision-making in high-intensity situations.) These jobseekers are aware of the potential for hiring bias but don't know how else to explain a career gap, or they figure care is such a part of their identity and employee needs that it's better to bring it up right away.

Other Millennials take it further: after having their eyes opened by living caregiving firsthand, they've observed a societal need and pivoted to caregiving- or eldercare-related careers. I've seen adults in their thirties who witnessed the poor treatment of ailing loved ones and chose a career in elder law to contribute to the protection of this vulnerable demographic. At a national caregiving conference, I met a young woman who is a licensed therapist. After her care experience, she decided to focus her professional skills on providing support to other caregivers and their emotional needs.

There are some high-profile examples in our generation: When her mother was diagnosed with early-onset Alzheimer's at age fifty-five, Lauren Miller Rogen, and her husband actor Seth Rogen, began Hilarity for Charity (now HFC), an organization that addresses Alzheimer's awareness and support for family caregivers of this disease. HFC has raised millions of dollars to grant in-home care and respite for family members and offers a free online caregivers conference annually.[17]

Alexis Ohanian, venture capitalist and cofounder of Reddit, has invested heavily in elder tech; he also champions paid leave and is a vocal advocate of paternity leave. He utilized the benefit himself when his wife, Serena Williams, nearly died after childbirth and he needed to be home to care for her and their newborn. He is also an investor in Papa, an app to connect seniors with young adults for companionship, transportation, and light tasks. Founder and CEO Andrew Parker created the app to help support his own aging grandfather.

IN THE SAME WAY IT'S A DISSERVICE TO VIEW SOMEONE SOLELY THROUGH the lens of their caregiving without taking into account all aspects of their self, we can't fully comprehend our care work without evaluating it in light of our career and economic landscape. Our economic reality has shaped different expectations and standards for our careers, and our families' need for care bleeds into that. Millennials intimately know the need for paid time off for family care and want a work environment that doesn't supersede every other part of our lives. We understand the intersection between care and capitalism—for better and for worse.

CHAPTER 18

WE'RE PAYING FOR IT: THE CARE COST CATASTROPHE MILLENNIALS CAN'T AFFORD

I know I'm not the only one who chose "Well, okay, I'll be poor, I guess, because I'm gonna take care of my mom."

—Brandon, 40

THE ECONOMIC FALLOUT OF THE PANDEMIC—SWEEPING JOB LOSSES, product shortages, and rising costs—brought into focus and the general discourse the economic standing of our generation. The bottom line: we were in trouble today, maybe worse trouble tomorrow. Personal finances worsened, savings dwindled, and credit card debt compounded. All this at a time in our lives when we might be hoping to buy a house or contribute to savings for a kid's college fund. Instead, savings (if we had any) were dipped into and housing was on the line. Like many things, the pandemic didn't create this problem: it illuminated the issue and intensified it—for everyone, particularly for caregivers.

The costs of care and everything associated with it liquidate our financial foundation even further. This can be true for any caregiver, yes—providing care isn't only emotionally taxing and time-consuming but also freaking expensive in dollars and cents and credit card swipes. But for our generation, care expenses can be detrimental in light of the other costs our generation has paid.

In 2019, a New America study on Millennial wealth stated: "Young adults in America today are on a much lower trajectory in their wealth accumulation than their predecessors. Dramatically so."[1] *Dramatically so.* The typical Millennial that year held 41 percent less wealth than a similar-age adult in 1989. In 1989, us older Millennials were big enough kids to look up at our parents and their friends and assume we were in for the same financial cushion; or, if our parents and the adults around us weren't doing so well, there were models out there to let us know we could be the generation to do financially better. It was messaging we were told…but for many of us, it hasn't worked out that way. At least not yet. (Economic predictions for the future aren't so good, either, but I'm an optimist—and caregiving has taught me, good or bad, you never know what's down the pike.) We're already familiar with reasons the Millennial generation is financially slammed as it is, but let's peel back another layer.

THE MILLENNIAL WEALTH GAP IMPACTS US ALL, ESPECIALLY CAREGIVERS OF COLOR

As mentioned, Millennials have spent the majority (or, for the youngest of us, *all*) of our employment history in a job market hit by major economic lows. Remember what we've already discussed about young adults in a recession: those who enter the job market at that time are compromised career-wise and financially for at least a decade. Whereas older adults were able to financially recoup after the Great Recession of 2007, in 2019 young adults still "lagged behind."[2] The situation hit people of color particularly hard. That New America study shares this insight:

> *Wealth gains made by Black and Hispanic families over the preceding decades were largely wiped out and have been slow to recover, which has amplified historic inequities and created new sources of inequality. As a result, the overall racial wealth gap has not narrowed over the last 30 years. The gap remains a chasm. Given the increasing diversity of the Millennial*

generation—one of its most salient characteristics—the racial wealth gap is clearly exacerbating the Millennial wealth gap.[3]

Simply, this post-recession wealth gap affected our entire generation but exacerbated another gap *within* our generation along racial lines. This was followed by another recession in 2020.

This is all important context when we talk about Millennials in caregiver roles: considering the racially diverse makeup of our generation, this wealth gap informs the financial picture of those who were already providing care before the pandemic as well as those who began caring then or after—before even taking care costs into account. The takeaway: Millennials are on the bottom end of a growing wealth gap, and when we consider this in light of how expensive caregiving is, we also need to take the diverse racial makeup of our generation, and our caregivers, into account.[4]

Student Loan Debt

Millennials account for almost half of outstanding student loan debt.[5] In dollars and cents, the average Millennial borrower has an outstanding loan balance of over $42,600. That's more than the annual income of at least a third of Millennials who are providing family care. Student loan debt is regularly cited as one of the primary factors Millennials have pushed off "life milestones" like having a wedding or buying a home.[6] It's a high price for education that can take a decade or more to repay. Brandon told me that when he stopped working to care for his mom full-time, his student loan debt interest was compounding to make his payments over $800 a month. "I'm paying hundreds of dollars a month to not be able to go anywhere," he said.

The Pandemic Knocked Caregivers onto Our Financial Asses

It's not a surprise that a global pandemic had terrible financial repercussions and threw us into another recession. Our country had the highest unemployment rate since the Great Depression.[7] Like I mentioned earlier, young adults were more susceptible to job loss during the pandemic; Black and Latinx Americans were also hit particularly hard. The situation for American women was so bad, a Bloomberg headline announced, "A Decade's Worth of Progress for Working Women Evaporated Overnight."[8] Women accounted for over half the job losses. One of the reasons women took the brunt of it: family care. More than 60 percent of workers said during the pandemic that their employer did not change policies to offer more flexibility for childcare or caregiving, and it was often women who were leaving the workforce to fill the roles at home full-time.

Many Americans didn't feel financially prepared for the pandemic.[9] Savings (for long-term goals, emergencies, or retirement) took a major hit. In normal times, the ages thirty through forty-nine (which a lot of Millennials were at the time) are considered "high-spending years" when expenses often rise faster than savings, including emergency savings, can keep up with.[10] The added pandemic effects weren't kind: by July 2021, a third of Americans said they had less money saved than before the pandemic; one in four had no emergency savings.[11] People overwhelmingly had less confidence in their financial future.[12]

TAKING THIS INTO ACCOUNT, MILLENNIALS ARE THE FIRST GENERATION expected to be financially worse off than their parents. Our finances have always stood on shaky ground because of bleak economic outlooks and opportunities—not lack of initiative—while our financial mobility has been unfairly compared to previous generations' without context. (In practice, we're actually a lot thriftier than our parents, and Gen Z, who grew up in the economic and housing shitshow, is proving even thriftier than us.[13]) Now let's add health care into the mix. Before the pandemic, the cost of care in our country was already exorbitant and could easily lead to personal bankruptcy, not to mention the cost of health care is greater for our generation. Unable to afford it, Millennials cut back spending on their own wellness activities. More than 60 percent couldn't afford preventative care.[14] In 2019, nearly half of

Millennials had put off medical or dental care that they needed for the same reason.[15] An emergency surgery could put someone into personal bankruptcy.

Caregivers are intimately familiar with medical expenses. Even financially challenged Millennials take on out-of-pocket costs for someone else's care, so the personal bankruptcy may be theirs. I want to clarify that this is *not* a result of youth or naivete: even AARP's national caregiving expert, Amy Goyer, shared how she declared personal bankruptcy because of her caregiving.[16]

Millennials in the caregiver role are vulnerable to a slew of costs.

OUT-OF-POCKET EXPENSES

Millennials pay more out-of-pocket costs for caregiving than other generations—on average, 27 percent of our income.[17] What's that in dollars and cents? The caregiving costs for Millennials totaled an average of $6,800 a year before COVID, but caregivers reported spending more per month since the pandemic's start.[18] Millennials also earn, on average, less than older generations yet make out-of-pocket purchases at similar or higher rates than they do. Long-distance caregivers may feel insecure that they provide "less" care because they are not always able to be physically present (we went over this; it's not true) but (in general) have more of a financial strain, paying almost double the out-of-pocket costs. (Dementia caregivers also pay significantly more than the average.)

What, exactly, is this money being spent on? AARP broke down the care costs incurred by Millennials as follows.

Household Expenses

About half of Millennials' caregiving expenditures goes toward household expenses. This includes rent or mortgage payments, home modifications, food purchases, and transportation costs. Household expenses are a higher share of out-of-pocket costs for Millennial caregivers than for other generations.[19]

Caregiving-Related Legal Costs

Caregiving-related legal costs are next on the list of our care expenditures. When you assume care for someone, there's legal paperwork that needs to be put into place: a will, a living will, power of attorney.... Lawyers prepare this paperwork, and it costs money. Legal costs are a higher share of out-of-pocket expenses for Millennial caregivers than for other generations.

Caregiving-Related Travel Costs

Caregiving-related travel costs are also a higher share of out-of-pocket expenses for Millennial caregivers than for other generations. When I was living in Los Angeles and traveling back to New York to be with my dad, either for a planned visit or a medical emergency, I was paying for cross-country flights. These aren't cheap to begin with and purchased last minute the prices skyrocket.

Caregivers may need to travel for reasons other than long-distance caregiving, too: Casey said that when she and her husband had exhausted the doctors and specialists in their area and still no one could provide answers about his chronic illness, they began to travel farther for medical care. Some of these appointments can now be taken over Zoom, but if not? You pay transportation to get there and for a place to stay.

Medical Costs

Medical costs can include co-pays and prescription drug costs. Recently, at CVS I overheard the guy next to me, a few years my junior, as he was picking up a prescription for his mom. When the pharmacist told him the cost after insurance, he was floored. Flipped out a little, even. And I get it, he was running a simple errand and it ended up costing him over a hundred bucks. Quickly, he resigned to the charge. "Well," he said, "it's not like her condition is changing anytime soon." He handed over his credit card.

These are just drug costs (and a hundred dollars isn't even close to how bad it can get). Depending on the illness or condition of the person you care for, a slew of treatments and therapies may be necessary to maintain their condition or improve it: physical therapy, speech therapy, and behavioral therapy are a few examples. Someone may also need to purchase adaptive clothing and accessories (like a shower rail, tub chair, adaptive cutlery), adult diapers, vitamin supplements. . . . Insurance can cover some of these costs, but not all. Sometimes it'll cover a specified number of physical therapy sessions, but when more are necessary to the person's longevity, what do you do? Other times, insurance covers physical therapy and speech therapy, but not in tandem: it's one or the other at a time. Walk or swallow. Medical costs (and there are a lot) constitute a relatively smaller share of Millennial caregivers' out-of-pocket expenses than for other generations, but they are still significant at 13 percent.

Somewhere on this list falls the cost of a nurse or home health aide—and they are freaking expensive. I've shared with you stories of caregivers who chose to keep their loved one at home (instead of in a nursing facility), but it was only possible with the help and care of an aide, whether part-time and supplemental, full-time while the caregiver is at work, or around the clock. It's also not unheard of for someone living in a facility to hire the additional part-time care of a private aide; it's a cost I took on when my dad was in the nursing home and I felt it positively impacted his quality of life there. As of 2019, the average cost of a part-time caregiver was $48,000 per year[20]—yes, that's just part-time. And the cost is understandable: you are entrusting someone with the life of someone you love who is medically vulnerable; it's a big responsibility. It's a lot of trust.

Kaci knew she'd only be able to manage caring for her mom at home *and* keeping her job by sending her mom to a day program and hiring a home aide. Medicaid pays for the day program for a certain number of hours per week, but the aide agencies that Medicaid covered, Kaci said, were terrible. People suggested options or told her about a great aide they had hired, but they all had something in common: they were privately paid for. Kaci couldn't afford an aide out of pocket, it was too much on her schoolteacher's salary; she also couldn't afford not to work. Eventually, her mom switched into the New York State Medicaid Consumer Directed

Personal Assistance Program (CDPAP), which pays for aides that patients are allowed to hire and fire on their own, outside of designated agencies. Though it's taken some trial and error to find someone who regularly shows up and that her mom gets along with, they have an aide now that, Kaci says, "has been awesome."

The key here is that Kaci's mom was eligible for Medicaid and that CDPAP allowed them autonomy. A lot of families in need of aide service are not as lucky. Also, people might (mistakenly) believe that Medicare pays for long-term care, like aide services or a living facility. Although people who have their own personal long-term care insurance are usually covered, the Medicare program for our nation's elders does not cover these costs—it's Medicaid that pays once you run out of money. While thank God Medicaid pays, it forces anyone with substantial (or even adequate) savings to "pay down" what they worked their lives for until it's gone, and with long-term care costs in this country as they are, a life's savings can go pretty quickly.

Also difficult is wrapping your head around Medicare and Medicaid benefits, understanding what different programs are available and if your loved one is even eligible. These long-term care programs and benefits often differ from state to state. Contacting your state's Office for the Aging can be the key to unlocking this knowledge. To my pleasant surprise, I've found state OFA websites are often chock-full of informative resources, and states like New York even offer a free helpline so you can speak with a professional who will answer your questions and walk you through.

Caring for Someone Financially Insecure

While Boomers are doing financially better than Millennials, they are doing worse than generations before them, with less home equity and total wealth.[21] For those of us caring for our parents, the age at which they retired didn't change but people are living longer off of the same retirement savings; funds are stretching thinner over a longer life span. Not to mention the recessions hit our parents, too, right in the retirement funds. The costs of co-pays rack up, and their insurance may not fully cover necessary medications, treatments, procedures, aides, or a live-in facility. We are left to pick up the slack.

One caregiver in her thirties said her parents did not save for their retirement. Her mother is now a widow whose health is in decline, so the young woman moved her mom in with her and gave up working during the pandemic to care for her. She has paid thousands out of pocket (just *in a single year*) for her mother's care. After acquiring significant student loan debt, she worked hard to get herself into better financial shape but now feels like it's all gone to hell. She's terrified that she'll end up in the same situation her parents were in but is at a loss for what to do about it.

"You're thrust into it [caregiving] and you may not even know what the care recipient's financial resources are," Christina Irving of Family Caregiver Alliance said. You might find that your loved one is strapped financially but has "too much" money to be eligible for Medicaid, so financial assistance seems completely out of reach.

But there is help out there. Without Medicaid, you may not easily (or at all) find financial support for long-term care, but identify other areas where you could use help, such as for food costs, utility payments, or medical devices not covered by insurance—there may be community resources or programs available with expanded eligibility, such as food pantries or discounted rates for medical devices, like a hospital bed. "Start with 'here are all the things that we're paying for that are difficult for me, is there help with any of these?' And then reaching out... You may try calling the local senior center and say, 'Do you have any information on public benefits or financial assistance programs for utilities, for groceries, for food?' They're going to know those programs and can probably give [you] some of that information. They may not be able to provide a lot of in-depth help... but they can at least maybe give some initial guidance." Irving also suggests reaching out to your county's Information and Referral services, a hospital social worker, or one community-based program that can help connect you to others.

The National Council on Aging suggests claiming the person you care for as a dependent on your tax return if they are eligible.[22] This allows you to deduct their expenses and utilize your flexible spending account (FSA) to pay for some of their medical supplies and appointments. Setting yourself up as your family member's legal power of attorney separates your personal expenses from theirs, which can protect you from being personally liable for their debts. Finally, working with a financial adviser can help you create a plan as well as enlighten you about care or medical programs your family may be eligible for. In an article for AARP, Amy Goyer shared that, in retrospect, she wishes she had found and utilized these programs earlier in her care journey.

Our Own (Crappy) Impacted Health

Caregiving is a stressor that negatively affects both our physical and our emotional health. You'll remember from earlier in this book, the lifestyle choices we make to cope (like alcohol, drugs) actually affect our mortality rate. In general, we are not in great shape (even if we look *good*) and, because of the economy, gave up gym memberships and preventative care. In short, we need therapy, medications, exercise, and to go to the doctor. These all cost money. Who's going to pay for all those cigarettes we're smoking? Just kidding, but who *is* going to pay for the deteriorating health we have as a result of caregiving? We are.

Loss of Wages and Social Security

I saved this one for last.

Millennials are more susceptible to employment interruptions as a result of caregiving. You'll remember that caregivers are often forced to miss days or weeks (or even months) of employment and, unless your company offers a care-inclusive policy, that time missed often goes unpaid. Some caregivers leave the workforce entirely, either planning to return later or pausing employment indefinitely. The missed work can total to days or years and creates a snowball effect: any loss of wages means less money paid into retirement plans and Social Security (which, for so many Americans, becomes a lifeline in older age).

The US Department of Labor's Women's Bureau by the Urban Institute studied women of our generation born between 1981 and 1985 and found that for those who have children and are also caregiving (either for a parent, parent-in-law, or partner), family care will cost close to $300,000 in lost wages, retirement savings, and Social Security over their lifetime. That's *each person*. The loss is 15 percent of lifetime earnings (think of the inequity in comparison to what a non-caregiver takes home). This was a higher lifetime cost of care than for men, but, as we know, men are not exempt. The study acknowledges these findings are likely conservative estimates; and compared with other caregiver studies, they are *very* conservative. Previously, a 2011 MetLife study of caregivers over fifty (so, Boomers) who care for an aging parent shows women to accumulate a total lifetime loss of wages and Social Security to be $324,044 from eldercare alone; for men it was $283,716. [23] As caregiving costs have since risen, we can believe the lifetime loss of wages and Social Security for Millennials will be worse—particularly for those who will be caregiving for decades.

You'll notice that working women (in general) face greater economic hardship because of caregiving. There are a few reasons why: When faced with care responsibilities, women are more likely to accept a less demanding job, give up work entirely, or lose job-related benefits in order to provide care. [24] The gender wage gap: if you're married and one of you needs to stop work to provide care, chances are the person who makes less money is the one who quits. Women who are single (which, we discussed, a lot of Millennial women are) who are caring for elderly parents are 2.5 times more likely than noncaregivers to live in poverty in old age.

Out-of-pocket care costs can potentially run you close to $1,000 a month; for those of us who are multigen caregivers also raising children, this is in addition to childcare costs, which, for an infant, run on average $1,300 per month. [25] Given the rising costs of eldercare, in our generation the out-of-pocket costs for caregiving are set to outpace the cost of raising children.

How exactly are we paying for these large additional expenses of family care? In a survey of multigen caregivers during the pandemic, almost 70 percent reported taking care costs out of their own daily budget.[26] Almost half were contributing less to their savings, and almost a third were contributing less to retirement. (Already we can feel the long-term implications brewing....) Twenty-seven percent took on more working hours to bring in extra income (reminder: they were already putting a significant amount of hours toward paid work and unpaid care), and the same percentage said they were drawing from emergency savings. People also reported paying off less debt to instead pay for care costs, delaying paying other bills, and taking on an additional job. Any one of these is not an option to be taken lightly. You can begin to wrap your head around how this could pan out to be a care cost catastrophe in our long run. It begs the question: How will we afford getting older ourselves? The situation is unsustainable and one many caregivers fear.

It Makes No (Business) Sense

We as families and individuals are not the only ones to suffer financially as a result of family care. In 2021, caregiving cost the US economy $44 billion in lost productivity based on work missed and the loss of more than 650,000 jobs to care. This was almost double the bill we faced ten years earlier.[27] Deteriorating caregiver health indirectly affected our economy in a significantly worse way, to the tune of nearly $221 billion in economic impact.[28] Caregivers are the human cost of our country's care and leave policies. Those who leave jobs to cover for care expose a national care infrastructure that protects businesses while hanging out to dry the working family members stuck filling a healthcare void and earning their own living and protecting their health.

GOOD NEWS (KINDA)

Central to this conversation about our generation's financial survival is the juggling act of earning income at a job while providing care without support or job protections available to do it all. Congress has yet to pass proposed bills and programs to expand family care compensation nationally. In the interim, most states have begun paying family caregivers an hourly wage, often through Medicaid, with eligibility and requirements varying by state.[29] For example, CDPAP in New York allows eligible patients to hire family or friends to provide their care; the program then pays the caregivers approximately $16 to $21 an hour.[30] This option has come up for discussion among Caregiver Collective members: some said they took advantage of their state's program; others said their state didn't offer it. Some said their family member wasn't eligible for Medicaid, which operates the program; others were denied because of their relationship (a spouse would be eligible, but not a girlfriend; in other cases, it's the other way around). One member said she utilized her state's program during COVID when it was too risky to bring in outside help, but then she'd transitioned out when she could because it was too taxing to provide care for her parents-in-law in addition to raising her kids and working in her own career.

Since 2022, Kaci has been paid to care for her mom through New York's CDPAP. Although her mother has been living at home with Kaci since 2015, Kaci was previously not eligible to be paid for care because it excluded daughters and sons from being paid. Finally, the eligibility standards changed. She said it helps but doesn't cover the extent of hourly care she provides.

"You have to have one aide with you, you can't do it all by yourself because it's so many hours. My mom qualifies for seventy hours. Really, I did the math, and I put in about ninety hours. With the aide service in addition." This was ninety hours of care in addition to her teaching career. Even being paid (thankfully), the balance is still difficult. Being paid for your family care is a solution for some, but not a fix for all or a solution to our country's larger care crisis.

PART FIVE

SOLUTIONS

CHAPTER 19

THE CHANGES WE NEED

KEITH ELLISON SAID, "THE WORK OF OUR GENERATION IS TO SAY GOOD-bye to old practices that don't serve us anymore." The Minnesota attorney general was referencing policing strategies in the wake of a guilty verdict for the murder of George Floyd, but his words are a good reflection of the times we're living in. Millennials are aware so many of our nation's problems, like systemic poverty and climate abuse, are the result of cycles that predate us. Our society debates sweeping reform for issues ranging from gun control to Confederate statues to catch up to what our reality looks like *today*; to face the problems that require our immediate action. The issue of family care should be no different.

"There's such a need for those larger systemic changes," Christina Irving said. "We have certain things, like the RAISE [Family Caregivers] Act, and there is a National Strategy on Supporting [Family] Caregivers now.[1] ... How is it *really* going to trickle down to where people actually feel the impact, where it is evident within services? I think we've seen a little bit more done within the Medicaid systems that have included enhanced caregiving supports, but it varies so much based on where you live."

When it comes to the big picture of family care in our nation, that last part Christina mentions has been one of the most eye-opening reveals to me in writing this book. Familiar with the resources I was able to access for my dad in New York City (albeit with research and creative thinking and sweat equity and personal funds and a mom who's a social worker), and informed on how cities often provide extensive eldercare and community services that smaller areas cannot, I was still shook by the differences in what my dad was able to access compared to what was available to other families in other areas of the United States; even in other areas of New York state. From speaking with caregivers across the country, and then following up with my own research of their state's policies, I've learned how much inconsistency there is when it comes to resource and support access. So much depends on where you live, so much depends on your peer group and whether you can afford private care. Resources are inequitable; accessing them is a disjointed process no matter where you live.

THERE ARE THREE SYSTEMS I SEE THE MILLENNIAL CAREGIVER OPERAT-ing within and at the mercy of: their place of employment, the healthcare system, and our federal government. I've listened (and continue to listen) to countless caregivers relay the obstacles they face, the stressors that take a toll on physical and fiscal longevity. Examining their issues within these systems that structure our lives and care, it's obvious: our societal frameworks are outdated and at odds with how our generation is living.

At a book-reading event not too long ago, I met journalist Evan Osnos. He asked me, in my opinion what was one solution to the caregiving crisis in our generation? It's a question I've been asked for years, so my answer was ready to go.

PAID FAMILY LEAVE

From the data I'd read to hearing the grievances of cash-strapped care-givers who had to take unpaid leave to provide care, either temporarily or indefinitely, it was the obvious solution. The fact that the United States doesn't have any sort of national paid-leave policy in place, I believe, is a massive embarrassment. I can argue up and down all day, with facts and figures, why our country needs a federal paid-leave policy that includes caregiving.

As time passed, my observations changed. I decided to informally poll the members of Caregiver Collective: In an ideal world, but given their current care situations, what "solution" would help them to balance it all? Paid family leave (PFL) to allow for time off work for care got a significant response. The overwhelming winner, however, was affordable in-home care that enables them to work full-time.

The poll illustrated a key point: caregivers want to work. We want ownership over our lives. We want to be there for family, we want to provide them care, but we don't want to do *only* that. We want to work toward our future, build and maintain stability, and still be there with the person we love who is ailing—knowing they are getting the quality care they need without us having to provide it all. We know from Jesus, who was eventually able to afford in-home care with his increased salary, that this is no cakewalk: you are still a caregiver, you are still reeling from the complicated health issues of someone you love; but you shouldn't have to devote, or even sacrifice, every ounce of yourself to do it.

That doesn't make paid family leave obsolete. Don't be mistaken, we need it, too. There will still be emergencies we must be present for, maybe some entail weeks or months of being bedside, and we should have the option of being there if that's what feels right. Other times, aides might call in sick or have an emergency of their own, and there will be lapses in paid care that need to be covered. In other instances, some people still choose to provide care for their family member full-time. My point is: *We should have choices in how we and our families receive care when they, or we, need it.* There is no single blanket solution. We need a reevaluation, not Band-Aids.

Addressing the big scope of providing care in our country, including caregiver needs, could be accomplished by a system referred to as "care infrastructure," which includes the policies, services, and resources that help meet family caregiving needs.[2] Paid family leave policies, community-based caregiver training, and access to affordable hired care all fall within a care infrastructure. It's important not only for the provision of care but to keep our society running: "The lack of care infrastructure affects our entire economy," a Biden White House fact sheet states.[3] Despite this, a care infrastructure is widely absent from US government. We need to ask *why*. What's the hurdle we need to overcome to get a functioning system of care moving?

TURNS OUT, THERE ARE A LOT OF HURDLES. SOME ARE PRACTICAL ISSUES, such as how to pay for particular care proposals; others are born of deeply ingrained biases on the value of care—and the value of those providing it. Not too long ago we watched this play out on the national stage.

CARE AS A FEMINIST (AND EQUITY) ISSUE

In the wake of the pandemic and its financial and health repercussions, President Biden released the American Families Plan and American Jobs Plan which addressed the caregiving crisis we'd just witnessed on full display. This "Build Back Better" agenda that was introduced to Congress packaged care as infrastructure necessary to the functioning and strength of our workforce and economy; it included plans for a national and comprehensive Paid Family and Medical Leave Program and expanding access to long-term care services under Medicaid, among other proposals. "The Biden administration and its allies are pushing the notion that caring for children—and the sick and the elderly—is just as crucial to a functioning economy as any road, electric grid or building," wrote the *New York Times*. "It's human infrastructure, they argue, echoing a line of thought long articulated by feminist economists (and often ignored)."[4]

The proposed programs instigated a fervor. One discussion topic hotly talked about in the news cycle was the controversy and debate around this question: *Is care work infrastructure?*

This was my Christmas. And also: *Oh, absolutely.* Our healthcare system relies on family care…providing this care directly affects the workforce and economy...how could the network of labor devoted to family care to keep our society afloat and alive *not* be infrastructure?

Despite a wide margin of bipartisan likely voters' support, the plans faced a lot of pushback both in Congress and in the media. For example, *Forbes* published an article titled "No, 'Infrastructure of Care' Is Not Infrastructure—and Three Reasons Why It Matters," which enumerated why the writer, Elizabeth Bauer, believed using the word *infrastructure* to refer to care was inaccurate and convenient misappropriation to further a political agenda.[5] One reason: the "redefining of words" such as *infrastructure* is an ethical breach employed by advocates "to persuade others to support their cause, by presenting data and sound arguments." "How am I to believe the statistics they present to me," Bauer wrote, "if I know that they are willing to engage in this sort of redefinition of terms to suit their political objectives?"

Oy vey. Articles like this are ridiculous, eschewing genuine societal need and the machinations of how systems fit together to function, and framing statistics as something "to be believed" rather than informed by. But this is what the "care as infrastructure" debate was under the influence of: political grandstanding born of opinions and outdated modes of thinking, rooted in traditional conservative notions rather than current actualities. (According to her bio, Bauer, an actuary and *Forbes* senior contributor, has an MA in medieval history, the application of which, as I see it, may have informed her opinion.) It wasn't just medievalists: as care maven (and Gen Xer) Ai-jen Poo pointed out, "*Politico* went so far as to say that it's 'silly' to call care infrastructure."[6] Ultimately, the debate in Congress hit an impasse and the infrastructure bill only passed once caregiving was removed.

This vocal pushback (by some) on accepting care as necessary for our nation's operation was the concept's most recent objection, but not its first. In a 2021 *New York Times* opinion piece, Anne-Marie Slaughter reminded us that this debate is rooted in decades-old sexism. The longstanding argument, made by feminist theorists and economists alike, points out that because family care has traditionally been deemed "women's work" and long gone unpaid or underpaid (whether by stay-at-home mothers or the many women of color working in care), its contribution is undervalued. *It's just what women do*, a role fueled by love and not dollars. As long as that notion is ingrained in men who benefit from this unpaid work *and* legislate, care will never be valued as the buttress to society that it is. As Slaughter wrote:

> *Insisting that there is actually a fixed definition of what infrastructure is—bridges, but not baby care—perfectly encapsulates the ways in which the world is still shaped by men. Not just conservative men, but men across the political spectrum. Men today, that is: Three-quarters of a century ago, the Greatest Generation recognized that both forms of infrastructure were essential to the war effort.*[7]

The title of her article, "Rosie Could Be a Riveter Only Because of a Care Economy. Where Is Ours?," is a reference to previous federally subsidized care support: during World War II, the US federal government funded universal childcare through the opening of federally subsidized day care centers, with the purpose of driving women into the workforce where they were needed to work wartime jobs.[8] So eighty years ago, the US government recognized, and supported, family care providers participating in the workforce, but now...?

These conversations were not only happening during the pandemic and are not only heard in policy circles. In my conversation with Dr. Ranak Trivedi, the researcher at Stanford University, about the lack of institutional medical system interventions to alleviate caregiver stress, she raised this point: "Part of the reason caregiving is both undervalued and all these things are underappreciated is because it's primarily women...caregiving is a women's rights issue, it's a feminist issue, and it's a women's health issue."

LACK OF CARE INFRASTRUCTURE, OR CONSIDERATION FOR INCLUDING care as an element of our nation's overall infrastructure, drives societal inequity. By dictating who is "allowed" to participate in the workforce or how many hours they can work in light of home care needs, caregiving of course creates a financial hit to those providing it—we've detailed that in previous chapters. It's not a leap to understand how this drives inequity in our country between those who provide care and those who don't—or haven't yet. "If the status quo [we experienced during the pandemic] continues, it will cleave the post-pandemic economy into two classes of workers: people with caregiving responsibilities and everyone else," Melinda Gates wrote in a 2020 *Washington Post* article, referencing words spoken to her by Adrienne Schweer of the Bipartisan Family Center.[9] Because of the history of who provides care in our country, and taking into account the gender wage gap, women are disproportionately affected by lack of care infrastructure. According to the White House, "Research shows investments in the care economy would increase employment, especially for women, reducing the gender employment divide."[10] This doesn't even yet take into consideration the implications along racial divides and economic classes.

Care infrastructure has the power to improve equity, to pull our generation out of a deep fiscal hole and give us a chance at economic recovery. What's occurred recently in this debate around care as infrastructure demonstrates that not everyone is ready to embrace (or even provide) the changes we need, but likely bipartisan support from voters is there.

WHAT WE NEED IS A LANDSCAPE AND POLICIES THAT MEET US WHERE WE are. How can these systems—place of employment, the healthcare system, our federal government—evolve to support the caregiving our society relies on, that our families depend on? The following chapters explore this question. We won't get into every policy or program in existence, even some that came up frequently in conversations with caregivers and caregiving experts (like how screwed up it is that our country necessitates "spending down" your financial assets to be able to receive Medicaid benefits for long-term care). Instead, in each chapter we will focus on an issue that Millennial caregivers experience and the ways it might make sense to address it.

These "solutions" are based on my observations, the conversations I've had, the research I've reviewed, and what caregivers themselves have told me. While considering ways we can reshape our systems to enable better care for everyone, I've realized: we already have some of these solutions in our sights, they are just not widely available or utilized. Sometimes putting these programs, or new ways of thinking about care, into action requires retraining our brains, a radical rethink. The radical rethink is not only for our systems but also for ourselves. If we are overwhelmed by care, how can we get the personal help we need—even if that means a break from our norm? Millennial caregivers are more likely than previous generations to ask for help, so let's explore and discuss some support solutions that can help us now and the generations to follow.[11]

CHAPTER 20

A BATH BOMB DOES NOT FIX THIS: SELF-CARE IS NOT THE SOLUTION

One of the most frustrating things I found during caretaking—well, I'd have to make a list to rank them—but when someone would say, "Don't forget to take time for you." And I was like, "Where do you expect me to find that time? I'm just so curious, what do you think I'm doing with it?" And I think it's obviously the most kind, well-meaning thing to say, but it just shows how there's absolutely no awareness, I think, around how much care goes into taking care of someone who's incapable of taking care of themself. Because it's like, "Well, should I not make breakfast? Because then my mom will starve. Or should I not wash the bedsheets after she has an accident? Because then she's gonna sleep in her pee. So what time should I make for myself?!" That just triggered me constantly.

—Alexandra, 33

Last year I was away from home, in Virginia, for the end of my uncle's life. We weren't yet sure it was the end. He had advanced Parkinson's and was on hospice care; weeks earlier my mom had received a call saying he had only a few days left, and the stress of it raised her blood pressure to a level so high that she needed to be hospitalized. EMTs worried she was about to have a stroke. My mom was admitted for a few days, until she was stable enough for us to leave to get to my uncle. The doctors didn't recommend her discharge but understood why time was of the essence. I drove us the seven hours to Virginia and we arrived to see my uncle had improved; he wasn't totally with it, but he was dressed, sitting up, and chatting a bit in the meal room. So when my mom got the call again, about a week after our return to New York, this time our deep concern was tinged with slight skepticism. Unwilling to take the chance, we packed up, arranged another rental car, and did the drive again.

My mom and aunt were my uncle's family caregivers. He also had the care of his hospice team and nursing home, but I still felt the stress deeply—okay, that's an understatement. That entire period—sitting with my mom while she was hospitalized, terrified I was about to lose another parent as I knew her; the multiple trips to Virginia within weeks for my uncle, the second trip which was the end; being by his bedside until he passed while we were getting dinner; then the quick succession of planning a funeral, going through his effects, and the need to be the logical, purpose-driven one because my mom and her sister were in such deep shock and grief at the loss of their brother—I was a fucking mess. The entire thing brought me back to my dad's disease and the day of his death and layered a new disturbed memory of trauma and grief on top of it.

I remember, while we were there, going for lunch at my favorite restaurant in Virginia, an old-timey diner with tabletop jukeboxes and wide pleather booths and oldies music and an extensive menu I love. Before this occasion, I'd spend the day before trips to Virginia for family holidays thinking about what I was going to order at the diner when we arrived; it's an experience I anticipate. This time, I didn't have the energy for it. I really felt like saying, "Please bring me *whatever*," and if it was something I'm allergic to, I'd just eat around it. Really, I had no capacity for thought or my own nutrition. But one thing I knew I did want: a Cherry Coke. I just wanted that so bad, the taste of something super sweet and fizzy to lift my mood. When it arrived, I pulled the straw from its paper and took a long sip, closed my eyes with relief. I could lose myself, for a moment, in that sip. Only looking back now do I realize this was my moment of self-care. It was all I could afford myself during that intense time, and it was exactly what helped—even if just for the duration of the meal.

Taking care of yourself and addressing your own needs, no matter how pressing the need, can be damn near impossible when everything else revolves around somebody else. Yet, every caregiver well-being resource refers to the need for self-care. It's always accompanied by the old adage "put on your oxygen mask first so you can help others." In this case, the oxygen mask is something like listening to music, calling a friend, going for a walk. (Or getting a Cherry Coke.) Caregivers often don't prioritize, or even address, their own feelings or needs and I understand the need for a reminder. Nevertheless, I call severe bullshit on this.

Millennials already know about self-care: the concept of our self-care is sold to us as the remedy for everything from a tough day at the office to regulating metabolism for brain function, and it's turned into (lucrative) commerce. So, when self-care is also the prescription doled out to alleviate the profound and chronic condition of caregiving, the suggestion rings hollow. Many don't even bother. Additionally, selling self-care as a caregiver's oxygen mask perpetuates the role of caregiver as servant to the healthcare system and the needs of their family before their own. It eliminates value for their well-being as a human and instead makes us a better functioning care machine operating on low battery instead of empty. And sadly, that's what convinces caregivers to heed the advice. *If you do this, you can get through another day!* The current approach to caregiver "wellness" puts total responsibility on us, and it's not a long-term solution for Millennials who will care long term.

And yet: yes, self-care is necessary. I'm talking about self-care as a means for managing your own well-being and resilience, especially in the face of care. (By *resilience*, I mean the Family Caregiver Alliance's definition: developing emotional skills for coping and stress and improving your ability to rebound from difficult situations.[1])

When it comes to self-care, research has shown that caregivers are, frankly, bad at it: in a study of relatives of patients with advanced cancer, all of them, no matter their reported level of "caregiver burden," were less likely to engage in self-care activities than the normative population.[2] Almost half of those with "high caregiver burden" said they hadn't been well-informed on how important self-care was, and it is: meditation, a self-care practice, has been shown to help balance the nervous system of family caregivers.[3] Less self-care in caregivers was found to be associated with poorer performance in providing care.[4] As Millennials, we have a leg up in our knowledge of self-care, but we also need to recognize how important it is within the scope of this particular care role and life experience. So, yes, I admit the reminder is necessary as is the need to communicate why.

Look, when you're utilizing effective methods of self-care like meditation or exercise, this stuff *works*. It helps to reduce stress, focus our thinking, calm anxious minds. I am a proponent. That study of advanced cancer patient families said caregivers

> *often restrict their leisure time and social time to meet the patients' needs. Some informal caregivers also tend to give priority to the patients' needs over their own. Clearly, when the patient's needs increase over time due to disease progression, relatives will even have less time available for self-care activities. This is worrisome as self-care activities are important for the well-being of relatives and for their ability to continue caregiving activities.*[5]

Here's where my grievance with caregiver self-care comes in: it is framed as a coping mechanism, something to do *to be a better caregiver.* Instead of helping ourselves to be of better service to others, I prefer to think of those L'Oréal commercials from the nineties: "Because you're worth it!" (Hair flip.) Here's the problem: it's *this* notion, the valuing of oneself, that is so often the hurdle preventing these young adults from taking even a few minutes just for themselves. Michelle felt guilty doing anything that wasn't work or care related; at times, that guilt led her to cancel plans with friends or abstain from socializing altogether. Not to mention (although Alexandra did) that your time is stretched between doctor appointments, researching treatments, going to work, helping your grandpa into his wheelchair and maybe your kids into their beds. Oh, and you need to sleep, too. Time and energy are limited. Caregiver care ends up not existing.

HOW AND WHY THE SELF-CARE RX FALLS SHORT

The self-care Rx not only falls short of addressing the scope and gravity of the issue but also undermines it. More than one member of my caregiver group felt so underwater that they expressed suicidal thoughts (remember the alarming rate of caregiver suicide ideation). The self-care conversation needs to take the onus off the *self* to be of benefit; these caregivers may not be seeing themselves clearly enough to understand what they need.

Care for the caregiver, I believe, requires outside help and services. For example, in 2015 New York governor Andrew Cuomo announced a $67.5 million grant to help ease the burden of informal dementia caregivers, which included money for counseling, support groups, and a twenty-four-hour hotline in addition to other services.[6] He wasn't the first: several other states had similar, smaller, programs already in place.

However, we can't only rely on others stepping up for our own well-being. In this chapter, I'm focusing on how caregivers can care for themselves in a lasting way—not as a way of letting outside intervention (whether from services or a friend) off the hook but as another piece of the puzzle, and one that can feel pretty empowering.

THE CARE CAREGIVERS NEED

When I asked caregivers what has helped them the most, or how they came to make an important decision in their own self-interest, they always had the same answer: **therapy**. Having been raised in a time when anxiety and depression were already part of the dialogue, we place less stigma around therapy. Millennials are more willing to talk about mental illness than our parents or grandparents were.[7] Debbie shared with me the importance of having a professional to talk to about dealing with her mom's dementia and care, the effect it has had on her life:

> I'm a therapist myself and I very much see the value in having someone non-judgmental to talk to you about all your emotions. And just sometimes those gentle reminders [that] you're human and it's okay that you feel this way. It

doesn't make you a bad person, a bad daughter. And I feel like I've person-
ally had that reinforced over and over throughout my caregiving.

Remember how Michelle was able to make care-related decisions, like deciding *not* to donate her kidney to her mother, by weighing them with her therapist? She thought that anyone in her personal life would be biased because of their relationships with her and her family, that their advice would not evaluate the situation objectively. She first sought therapy because she knew she needed emotional help; she didn't realize what she was looking for at the time was someone who had her back and kept Michelle's best interests in mind.

Dr. Feylyn Lewis spoke about the importance of talking to a professional who "understands the nuances of caregiving." In her research, she has seen the impact speaking to a professional, whether a therapist or a trained worker, has had on younger caregivers. "I've seen what a difference they make to young people in terms of being able to have that person outside of their family that they come talk to and turn to and vent and cry. And sure, happy moments too."

My advice: *Seek help before the situation becomes dire.* Alexandra told me that she wishes she had put therapy into place sooner, while she was still caring for her mom and not after. "But," she asked rhetorically, "where do you find the time?"

There are ways: online therapy is more available to us now and it's a tool caregivers say they utilize—especially because it's convenient. Caregivers are short on time, and teletherapy eliminates the time (and money) of travel. Even if you don't find the therapist perfect for you right away, take the step. It might take a little bit of trial and error, or it might be a stopgap until you are able to go in person, but taking the hour to get things off your chest helps. (Check out the back of the book for resources.)

Respite is another useful (although occasional) tool. A lot of caregivers come into the group not knowing what this word means. In short, *respite* is a short-term break. It can last an hour or a few days, and there are programs devoted to providing responsible care for your person so that you can get away, to get a haircut in peace or even to travel. Caregivers can apply for respite through various organizations, whether caregiving organizations or organizations associated with the disease or illness their family member is dealing with. Some hospitals even offer respite.

Kaci knows how difficult travel respite can be to plan. Even making the decision to leave on a trip can be difficult. But travel was a huge part of Kaci's identity, she said, and a thing she loves to do; once her mom moved in, seven years went by without Kaci taking a trip. She decided to plan a vacation with a friend to Vietnam, to take a break from the stress of care and work and to reconnect with her identity from "before." It would be the biggest trip she had taken in a while, and making the decision to go or not was stressful. I asked Kaci how she reached her decision.

"Therapy. That was a lot of it, her helping me work through those ideas and plans. Also, I had a friend who kind of pushed me in some ways, because she bought the ticket. We bought the ticket a year in advance, so I had a whole year to plan." She said the coordination was difficult because there's a lot of "power" that goes into preparing everything. She hired aides well in advance and installed security cameras so she could check in on her mom; she anticipated the times her mom would not pick up the phone because she was asleep or didn't hear it ring, so the cameras were an effort to eliminate Kaci's panic in advance. Not everything went smoothly while she was away: there were instances when aides didn't show up, so Kaci called her brother and told him, no excuses, you need to get over there.

"Getting breaks is helpful," social worker Christina Irving said. "How accessible that is really varies based on what public benefits they're eligible for, what community resources exist, where they live, whether they have family or friends that can step in and provide that help. Exploring that is important." A research study on caregiver burden and self-care cites respite care as a potential intervention to improve quality of life, but notes caregiver support needs are often unmet.[8]

CAREGIVERS USE OTHER POWERFUL SELF-CARE PRACTICES, TOO. WHEN I reached out to one caregiver, asking to interview her for this book, she had a definitive answer. Sorry, she replied, but she was finally learning to carve out time for herself. She was trying to place limits on how much time she spends thinking about caregiving.

I thought: *Good for her.* This caregiver is a great example of **setting boundaries**. Setting boundaries is not easy and requires getting comfortable with saying no. Caregiving can feel so all-consuming, I appreciated that she knew she didn't want to spend additional time discussing it.

Ron and Michelle also drew boundaries when they each made the decision to separate their personal living spaces from where they care, choosing to live on their own and no longer with the parent they care for. I had conversations with both of them during each of their decision-making processes as they considered whether it was even feasible. For both, the decision did not come easily or quickly—but eventually, they both realized having a separate living space from the care recipient would deliver the best outcome. Michelle met many obstacles in that quest, but she didn't give up. She persisted as an advocate for herself and eventually bought her own apartment. Though it took longer than she probably would have wanted, she did it, with the help of her dad, who accompanied her through the process, and a family friend, who spent time with her mom while Michelle and her dad went to the closing. Both people stepped up to help her get this done. There's a lesson in this: the more people you're honest with about the help you need, the larger your support network will be to help you.

Debbie was plagued by the idea of her mom living alone, always nervous something would happen to her. By moving her mom into assisted living, Debbie gave herself peace of mind and room for balance in her own life. It's a different version of setting boundaries, deciding to let someone else in on her mom's care. "She's in a higher level of care, she's receiving that support. I don't know...how long this part of life will be, but I've had to make my life more sustainable. Just to be there for her, to be there for my husband, and to be there for myself. To have a life that just feels more manageable and isn't a feeling like an uphill struggle all the time."

She said that since moving her mom into assisted living, she's realized she needs to take life less seriously and learn to have fun again. It's a process she's working on.

BRANDON TOLD ME HOW MOVING IN AND CARING FOR HIS MOM FULL-time increased her reliance on him; once she surrendered certain things (like when she began to let him help her into the shower), she began to depend on him for everything. One of the things he's been working on is reevaluating where other people can step in to address her needs. Similar to Debbie, Brandon said **outsourcing** has been helpful in alleviating (somewhat) the "struggle" of caregiving and maintaining his own well-being. He calls it "a constant negotiation . . . to re-look at, 'Okay, what do we really need me doing? And what can we outsource to someone else?'" One example: finding his mom a therapist and people to talk to has allowed the mom-and-son duo a needed separation.

Relieving some of your duties where you can is important: research has shown those with "high caregiver burden" were less resilient than the normative population, while relatives with less burden were more resilient than the normative population.[9] Alleviating how much care you take on—not doing it all—can be effective self-care.

JESUS, THE STAND-UP COMEDIAN, FILLED ME IN ON RESEARCH CONDUCTED by AARP and Google on what caregivers need most. The result: time, and **laughter**. According to the Mayo Clinic, laughter induces actual physical responses that alleviate stress and are good for our health (for example, we take in more oxygen when we laugh, which stimulates organs and increases endorphins).[10] Jesus had opinions on laughter's purpose in caregiving: "I think it services more than we're able to tell it in medical journals or medical books. I think it does more for us than we're able to tell right now."

NOT EVERYONE IS A STAND-UP COMIC, BUT THERE'S SOMETHING TO BE taken from the idea of **creative expression**. A national caregiving conference I attended passed out coloring books and watercolors that were sponsored by AARP. I wouldn't have thought to pick up this activity on my own, but the gift and its accessibility created a little fun. I remembered how simply painting or drawing with no goal in mind, just letting your mind drift, can be so relaxing and temporarily reset your brain.

CAREGIVERS EXPRESSED A DESIRE FOR **SUPPORT GROUPS** SO THEY COULD hear and learn from others dealing with a similar illness or situation. Support groups can offer great, practical, layman's advice—I learned about vitamin supplements that helped some people with PSP but that a doctor wouldn't recommend because their efficacy wasn't proven in clinical trials (one was CoQ10, by the way—we bought it). Even though you are seeking the help of others, finding a support group and dedicating yourself to attend meetings (whether virtual or in person) is itself an act of self-care. You don't even need to share if that's not comfortable for you because, when you find the right group, just listening can be beneficial.

In my talk with Dr. Feylyn Lewis, she mentioned peer networks as a "successful intervention" for caregivers. It was through Caregiver Collective that Feylyn and I connected, years ago, when she was one of the first members to join. "What you had done with caregivers is unite us, bring us together where we are, with people who understand and relate and get it," she said. "That's extremely powerful."

ALTHOUGH THE TOOLS MENTIONED IN THIS CHAPTER CAN HELP CARE-givers make improvements in their lives, I want to leave you with this: Doesn't a constant SOS indicate a bigger problem, a broken system? Shouldn't we aim for a healthcare approach that doesn't exact such a toll on caregivers, rather than bandaging us up enough so we can get back out there? When we are having a conversation about care—how we treat people in our society—we should be evaluating, and accountable for, the care extended to everyone.

CHAPTER 21

HOW OUR *WORKPLACE* CAN HELP US (AND THEMSELVES)

I HAVE BEEN LUCKY ENOUGH TO HOLD REALLY COOL JOBS IN SERVICE OF building a writing career; getting a job on a TV show is not easy and staying in one is even harder. I loved it. But when my dad was hit by a health emergency when I was at work, I instantly did not give a shit about my office. In heightened moments like this, the priority comparison was a no-brainer. Over the long run, though, there's a choice to be made between long-term care and building a career. You remember you do give a shit about your job and, financially, you need it. Even holding a part-time job can be difficult when care needs are demanding. Think about all the caregivers we've heard from in this book and the myriad ways straddling work and care affects them.

As it was with maternity leave not too long ago, it may be up to workplaces and businesses to lead social change (I'm paraphrasing Bishop Michael Curry here). Private companies and nonprofits were forced to figure out maternity leave (I'm generously including those companies that require pregnant women to file for disability), but caregiving, for the most part, has not received the same treatment. Just as we won't stop having babies, we won't stop caring for aging, ailing, or disabled family members either—the number of caregivers will likely only increase. We need to respond to the work-care imbalance.

Some potential solutions are already out there, both on a national scale and on the corporate level. Still, far from every caregiver is covered, and at times, if taking days away from the office is covered, those days are unpaid. Remember Michelle, who took advantage of the Family and Medical Leave Act—twice? FMLA is great for job security, allowing twelve weeks leave within a twelve-month period, but that time away from work is unpaid. When some workers hear that, they decide not to utilize the benefit because they can't afford the missed paychecks. Also, FMLA only covers companies with fifty or more employees: remember Chelsea, whose employer threatened to fire her if she didn't return to the office from caring for her dad, who'd had a stroke? The law office Chelsea worked for was small, she was not covered by FMLA, so she didn't have any care leave benefit—paid or unpaid.

What Chelsea did have was someone willing to help her advocate for herself: a paid family leave advocacy group offered to coach Chelsea on how to approach her employer to petition for a change in benefits offered; basically, to make the case for why the company should offer time off for caregiving. This advocacy work has a good track record in winning paid leave for employees; it also addresses a need employers have a hard time denying: in a survey, 82 percent of employers agreed or strongly agreed that over the next five years caregiving would become an increasingly important issue for their company.[1]

After speaking with so many working caregivers and advocating for years for a national paid family leave policy, I'm going to discuss two strategies I believe employers can undertake to support their workers who also balance family care: offering care benefits to employees, and creating a "culture of care awareness."

OFFERING CARE BENEFITS TO EMPLOYEES

We can look to corporate examples that showcase how Millennials' family choices are already changing the workplace. These can give us a look at what the future of the workplace could be. Major corporations, such as

Coca-Cola, have already enlisted the feedback of their Millennial workers to remain competitive in recruiting and retaining young talent.[2] They found the ability to balance family care with their job was on the list of these employees' priorities and instituted policies to support it.

Workplace policies can be implemented to enable more employees to retain their jobs while also handling care responsibilities—for the companies that have already introduced them, they work. The areas the policies target? Caregiver-employee absenteeism, stress, isolation, and illness. These policies include flexible work hours, on-site or near-site childcare (also eldercare), caregiver referral services, and remote work (although it's important to remember this may not be possible for many service jobs and essential jobs, which are often lower paid). As we returned to offices after the lockdowns, some businesses decided to make work-from-home a permanent policy, although a portion of these companies quickly backtracked on this commitment. Policies like flexible work hours and remote work have been shown not only to help the caregiver but also to benefit the company: research by Harvard Business School shows company caregiving benefits and policies improve employee retention and have a good return on investment in dollars and cents.[3] Smaller companies might argue that they don't have the same resources larger corporations do, and they're right; but even small companies can offer care resources like support groups, paid sick days that can also be used for care, caregiver resource lists, and in-house stress reduction programs.[4]

Employee retention and corporate competitiveness as results of these care benefits aren't just stats on a chart. I've heard the human side of these situations discussed in Caregiver Collective. After Jessica, who cares long distance for both her parents and takes regular trips to visit them, earned her master's degree while working full-time and caring, she felt it was time "to move on professionally." She had been with her company for eleven years and wanted to work somewhere that offered more growth potential, but her current employer allowed flexibility and paid time off for care, and she wasn't confident she could find that elsewhere. "They had always been understanding and flexible with me, but career-wise I was just really stuck." She found a new job and it even gave her a raise, but the company was far less flexible around care. After four months, she returned to her previous employer.

CORPORATE CULTURE OF CARE AWARENESS

Here's a rough truth: even when care policies are offered, employees may not use them. This boils down to two reasons: either employees don't know these benefits are available, or they believe there is a negative stigma attached to using them. Creating a corporate culture of "care awareness" can help solve both issues and get people utilizing the support offered.

Some employees don't seek out or utilize their company's care benefits ("even if they are struggling"[5]) because they don't identify as a "family caregiver"—see how that identity piece creeps back in and why awareness is important? Not identifying as a caregiver negatively affects you in the workplace, too.

"It's important to use the term 'family caregiver' and help people understand they are caregivers," stated Susan Reinhard, senior vice president and director of the AARP Public Policy Institute, in AARP's Practical Guide for Employers.[6] This is part of building your company's culture of care awareness. Another aspect: educating employees on what care benefits are available to them. More than half of respondents in the AARP and Northeast Business Group on Health (NEBGH) survey of employers said employees were "not very" or "not at all" aware of caregiving benefits their company offered. So, that's cool. I hate to put something else on caregivers' to-do lists, but if you need advice or support on how to manage your job with your care responsibilities, check to see whether your company offers care benefits that you are unaware of. AARP suggests asking your Human Resources or benefits department or your direct manager for help so that you don't have to figure it out on your own. Companies building a culture of care awareness can help an employee realize they are a "caregiver" and can also help reduce (or eliminate) negative stigma employed caregivers may face or fear.

Therein lies our next problematic scenario: your company offers care benefits, you are aware of them, but you feel uncomfortable utilizing them. Remember how many people in our generation don't discuss their caregiving with supervisors or colleagues? There can be real fear around being looked down on or penalized if you need a day of leave for care. Think about Casey, whose boss "didn't know what to do with her"; and Ron, who felt coworker knowledge of his home experience would create a disconnect with peer colleagues. This fear may be validated externally or it might only be internal, but either way it can hold us back. Prepandemic research revealed that, "while 65 percent of employers said they offered flexible working arrangements—the most common caregiving benefit— only 39 percent of employees said they have used the benefit. Workers who haven't said they feared that a flexible work arrangement would make them seem less committed."[7]

Policies people don't use help no one. Reducing the stigma and giving employees the freedom to utilize caregiver benefits without fear begin with a company adopting a culture of care awareness.

So How Can a Company Do This?

It can start with a top-down approach. One study found "while employees hear their employers proclaim that they are concerned about their colleagues' caregiving needs, they do not see management 'walk the talk.' Instead, employees observe the apparent reluctance of senior management to use care benefits."[8] Company leaders need to be seen utilizing these benefits themselves. One high-profile example is investor and Reddit cofounder Alexis Ohanian, mentioned earlier. He took paid leave at his own company when he needed to care for his wife, Serena Williams, when she suffered medically after childbirth. As the boss, he was vocal that all employees should take this leave when needed.

Companies can also build care awareness by expanding the benefits offered to caregiving employees. Research indicates that the lack of company caregiver policies (in comparison to parental policies) could explain the difference in support for parents of young children versus caregivers of adult family members.[9] Companies can organize support groups for employees who are caregivers. New or young parents within a company find each other; they trade advice and support on managing their job with their parenting role. Caregiving should be no different. Finding each other within a single company can help build support, raise awareness, reduce stigma, and provide caregivers with an additional resource.

Finally, there's offering employees paid family leave that covers family care beyond childcare. Until there's a comprehensive federal program, if your state doesn't offer PFL, then employers are the next line of defense in protecting their employees when care needs arise. "Providing employees with some type of paid leave when caring for someone might be the single most important consideration for employers when thinking about creating a caregiving-friendly workplace," stated AARP in its Practical Guide for Employers.[10] "Some type of paid leave": not FMLA, not unpaid days off with the promise of not firing or demoting you, but the ability to take leave from the office without sacrificing your pay—so you actually take the days you need. You'd be surprised at how few companies offer this (or perhaps you're more realistic and won't be surprised at all): in 2023, just over one-quarter of civilian and private-sector employees had access to paid family leave from their employer;[11] the proportion of employees with access to unpaid leave was 90 percent or higher (remember, employees with access to PFL may also be granted unpaid leave through FMLA).

Meanwhile, business leaders can continue to pressure Congress to enact national paid family leave on behalf of their workers and themselves. In 2021, nearly two hundred business leaders came together to publicly urge Congress to create a "permanent paid family and medical leave policy."[12] Signatories included Airbnb's chief strategy officer Nathan Blecharczyk, Alexis Ohanian, and then-COO of Thinx Shama Amalean Skinner—all Millennials who understand the value of care and of the people they employ.

In this discussion of how few workers are covered by PFL, we also need to consider those who are self-employed or who own their own business. As of this writing, no existing state paid-leave programs automatically cover those who are self-employed (such as freelancers and independent contractors).[13] Instead, twelve of the fourteen states with existing state-run paid-leave programs (reminder: we have fifty states, so that's cool) allow self-employed individuals to voluntarily opt in by applying, adhering to the rules, and paying into the state's insurance system.[14] That leaves behind a lot of our country's self-employed workers (and remember how Millennials tend to make ends meet by starting their own businesses or participating in the gig economy).

The ability to take time off from work, and whether this is something an employer allows for, is a topic that has come up in Caregiver Collective with an additional point: aside from caregivers needing the time to provide the actual care, many Collective members also noted the need for the time and space to counteract caregiver burnout. Those who were not "regularly" employed had more flexibility to make the decision to take this time to reset, though still with repercussions: Faye had just started her own business when her mother's progressing dementia coincided with the pandemic. She said she felt like she was spinning her wheels, exhausted and depressed. After consulting with her husband, she decided to end her business. After some time, she noticed a "huge difference" in her well-being, feeling "more grounded, rested" without having to focus on so many things. Beck, whose life partner has a disability and requires care, has also taken periods without working. "Sometimes just focusing on caregiving has restored my strength and peace and I highly recommend it."

These caregivers aren't on vacation, they're providing care full-time without a paycheck or business ownership. Paid-leave programs could keep caregivers like them in the workforce by providing the days or weeks off necessary to provide care, or the space for them to reset and combat burnout.

CHAPTER 22

HOW THE *HEALTHCARE* SYSTEM CAN HELP US

L AST NOVEMBER, I WAS IN NEW YORK VISITING MY MOM FOR THANKS-giving. While in the midst of buying groceries and picking up the turkey, she got sick. *Really* sick. I took her to urgent care for what we assumed was the flu but which quickly escalated to her being sent to the ICU and a weeks-long hospitalization. Multiple medical teams were involved in her treatment: infectious disease, surgical, pulmonary...they raced to stabilize her, they raced to figure out what the hell she had and how she could have contracted it. I had seen my mom in the hospital before, but I had never seen her look like this. I was very literally sick with worry: I had frequent sudden dizzy spells and moments when I'd lose vision only to have it fade back in seconds later and I'd keep going. Finally, her condition went from stable to improved; she had color back in her face. We were told she would be discharged, thanks to the Almighty and the infusion therapy she'd receive at home three times a day for the next month.

Guess who'd be administering this IV medication? Yours truly, I was told. Ms. Squeamish with Needles and Blood was anointed her new at-home nurse. Chronic weeks-long stress over my mom getting better, surviving, had a moment's relief before I developed a new anxiety over handling this medical treatment myself. It was a fortunate scenario, of course, and we were lucky she would fully recuperate, but...oy.

My mom was discharged in the early evening, we arrived home to find large boxes of supplies and refrigerated medicine vials had already been delivered. At eleven that night, a nurse came over to instruct me on how to administer the infusions. I was grateful for the immediate professional handhold; I was also *tired*. It was a long day and late at night to be learning something so outside of my comfort zone and that involved a tube leading directly to my mom's heart. But there was no time for a timeout; my mom couldn't miss a dose, the medication regimen needed to kick into full gear right away.

Over the next weeks, I set alarms for three times a day so I could prep the drugs, then another alarm so I didn't forget to actually administer them. The schedule of treatments dictated my day. At some point, the steps became so easy and rote that at times I'd blank out and forget what I was doing. One time I remembered to wash my hands but forgot to wear the latex gloves and then freaked out that I'd somehow infected my mom; her nurse would get phone calls from me, panicked. While it may not have been as intensive and invasive as some home care can be, it was a lot for me.

WHERE IS THE SUPPORT?

During the weeks my mom was hospitalized, no counseling was offered to her or to me, the family member who was there every single day. A hospital chaplain visited her bedside, and from him she received spiritual support; his visits were a help to her and a relief for me to see she had someone to discuss theories of life and spirituality with and get a psychological reprieve from the environment...but we never saw a hospital social worker. A social work student visited once while my mother was in the ICU: she stood there with a clipboard and wanted to know if we'd need a shower chair for home...weeks before we even knew when she'd go home. My mom was going through a traumatic experience, and I was going through a different one right beside her. We already know the mental health toll that care and hospitalization have on us, the risk of PTSD....Where the hell was the support?

I ask this not from fantasy or delusion about what a social worker is—when I was born, my mom was director of social work at the very hospital she was now a patient in. I grew up learning about her job counseling patients and their families through cancer and AIDS, I saw the rounds she made on annual Take Your Daughter to Work Days. So, where was that counseling now that she needed it?

I learned that in the years since, the field of hospital social work has taken a hard turn. What was once a career in psychological counseling has become a job of administering the patient's transition from hospital to home; social work is now offering a shower chair instead of psychological support (and, yes, my mom needed one—I don't want to undermine the value of receiving the supplies and equipment you do indeed need). And this shift didn't just happen in this hospital or even in this city: Feylyn, who lives with her mom in Tennessee, had a similar experience when her mom was hospitalized for a stroke. She agreed that it would be a relief to us caregivers if our family member was provided professional emotional support at the time of their trauma.

"I think having someone for the ill or disabled person to talk to also would help alleviate that, I hesitate to say 'burden'... on the caregivers for that emotional support," she said. "Because I certainly know that it's true that we, as caregivers, also shoulder when the ill or disabled person has to bend [from]... all that they're experiencing. We also tend to take that in." Feylyn makes a really good point: our loved one's need for emotional support has an effect on us that can be twofold: it is difficult to watch someone you love experience a life-altering health event, or an ongoing health issue, and know they need someone to talk to who can uplift them, but it can be too much when that person turns to us to support all their emotional needs when we're also in need of support. We should not be put in the position of acting as their therapist as well as caregiver; it is too much to take on, and frankly, you're probably not equipped. Counseling for both sides of the care relationship should be offered. (I do admit, though, in generational terms it seems our parents and grandparents are more reticent about speaking with a therapist; but many do, and these resources should still be available. The more visible emotional counseling is, the better the chance of normalizing it.)

From what I understand, the hard turn the field of hospital social work took occurred in the mid-1990s, when health care adopted "hospital to home," a practice to shorten hospital stays by discharging patients earlier so they can recuperate at home. Around this time, health care also shifted to family-centered care, which empowered the patient and their family to be more involved in care planning and decisions, and allowed for less hospitalization with changes like my mom being able to receive infusion therapy at home rather than spending another four weeks in a hospital bed. The profession of social work then began to focus, seemingly entirely, on putting the pieces together to arrange for that transition to home; somehow the pendulum swung too far. The family members who take on the responsibility of care aren't treated as a member of the care team but instead are given the message: "Here, you do it." In fact, research by the AARP Public Policy Institute found that family caregivers are often left on their own to provide "intense and complex care."[1] The healthcare system that hands off the "patient" offers few services to us, in training or emotional support, in order for us to handle the stress of an ill or disabled family member or the stress of our role. As one study on caregiver burden noted, "Unfortunately, the support for these relatives seems no common practice, as unmet health care needs are still prevalent in this population."[2]

Dr. Ranak Trivedi, the psychologist and researcher at Stanford University who specializes in family caregivers, doesn't believe the emotional health of caregivers is taken seriously enough by the medical field. She noted how a clinician may address a caregiver about their stress but then does nothing to actually help them: They might say, "'What you need to do is stress management.' 'Okay, then tell me how.' They don't have an answer," she said. "They're just like, go do stress management. That's not an intervention. You don't say, 'Go do chemotherapy'; you would set it up. You wouldn't say, 'Go do cardiac rehab'; you will put a referral in and you will make sure the cardiac rehab is done."

Because the medical system relies on caregivers, keeping an eye on our well-being and stability should not be our responsibility alone—as the self-care prescription has us believe. The medical system needs to stop undervaluing caregiver behavioral health and enact some interventions to prevent the harshest of the mental health repercussions. When I wrote about caregiver PTSD for the *Washington Post*, doctor friends immediately reached out, asking, "What can I do?" Some interventions for caregivers when a family member is hospitalized have proved to reduce emotional trauma on the caregiver, and I believe the willingness of healthcare providers to help is there.[3] What can these professionals provide to improve caregiver well-being and, hopefully, prevent them from becoming burned-out patients themselves?

My proposal is twofold: behaviorally, we need professional support and intervention; functionally, we need training.

LOOK OUT FOR US WITH A FAMILY-CENTERED CRITICAL CARE APPROACH

There are many proposals for caregiver support, and some programs are in place, but the need is widespread, varied, and dire. One direct solution for the stress and emotional health issues I've heard repeated by so many caregivers is focusing on what can be done to help caregivers during a family member's hospitalization. I believe we already know some of the answers; one is taking a "family-centered critical care" approach to health care. A family-centered critical care approach acknowledges "like the CCI [chronically critically ill], family members have distinct characteristics and needs during an episode of chronic critical illness." This approach "aims to simultaneously recognize the needs of the patient and family during critical illness."[4] In my most recent caregiving stint for my mom, her large medical team could have taken this approach and also addressed our emotional needs.

Provide Counseling

While my mom was hospitalized, her primary doctor was kind, attentive and chatted with me a bit on a human level. I was open about the distress I felt, but my confessions were limited to passing conversation; really, we needed him there to fill us in on what was happening to my mom. Counseling, whether provided by a social worker or another trained professional, could have alleviated some of the emotional stress I was experiencing; maybe it would have prevented the dizzy spells, I can't say for sure. In her research on young caregivers, Feylyn found having a trained professional to talk to was found to have beneficial value; she stressed the need for this support to be free or low cost.

Dr. Trivedi said the obstacle she sees is that there are not enough experts in the clinical setting who are trained in caregiver support, so it's often the doctor who might check in with the family member present. "We need to value people who are experts in it and not just keep telling our XYZ specialists that they're also supposed to be providing therapeutic support for caregivers." When I heard this, I thought aloud:

> It sounds like there should be more of a specialty of social workers or psychologists who are particularly attuned to caregiver needs and research around caregiving, emotional behavior.

"Absolutely," she answered. "Because otherwise…we're continuing to devalue it by saying, 'Oh, we can just train you. Here's a box of Kleenex.' A box of Kleenex is all you need, right?…We need structured programs for caregivers, to support caregivers, to assess them. Meaning: screen them, and then do something about when they screen positive [for depression or PTSD]."

Screen Caregivers for Psychological Issues, and Other Early Mental Health Interventions

Dr. Trivedi mentioned caregivers should be "screened." These screenings are a tool that helps health practitioners evaluate the caregiver for mental health issues; studies have found they proved helpful in identifying caregivers in need of mental health intervention. A study of family members of chronically critically ill persons suggests questionnaires or face-to-face interviews can be conducted quickly to screen for symptoms of depression, anxiety, and acute and post-traumatic stress disorders (all of these sound familiar?) and can help direct the family members (us) to needed resources and supports to "help us through the stress of critical illness." "Early psychological screening among family members of the critically ill can identify individuals who may benefit from interventions that prevent further psychological impairment. Screening family members for risk for psychological disturbances will enable critical care nurses to coordinate resources in order to prevent additional psychological harm."[5]

There are other ways healthcare providers can, and should, reach out to caregivers. The researchers at Case Western Reserve University who conducted the study just cited recommend that medical teams reach out early to build trust, reduce uncertainty, and provide emotional support and empathy.[6] A high state of anxiety was identified as a risk factor for developing PTSD, suggesting early psychological screenings of family members as a preventative measure. In addition to screenings, Dr. Trivedi believes caregiver supports should be provided as part of the healthcare system.

One more suggestion: a study in Australia found that writing in a diary in the ICU can reduce the risk of PTSD in family members.[7] This suggests "reflecting on the difficult situation in the intensive care unit and later sharing reflections with the patient... may protect against posttraumatic stress in relatives"[8]—although there was no effect found on depression or anxiety. Caregiver PTSD as a concept is more accepted today, but more research is required to truly understand it and which interventions can help.

THIS ALL SOUNDS VERY GOOD: BEING SCREENED, BEING ACKNOWLEDGED, and being offered the professional help we need before our mental health spirals to a dark(er) place. I want to stress: the need is for the medical system we are interacting with to observe the caregiver and their health, conduct assessments... and be accountable. When my father died, a hospital social worker quickly arrived and asked whether I would like a follow-up phone call to check in on me. I told them I had a therapist, but yes. Why not. Even immediately, I knew I could use the most support and people checking up on me that I could get. They never called. I was okay, I had other support to catch me, but what if I didn't? It hurts to imagine those who fall through the cracks.

So what's the holdup? We know this works, that it helps people, so why don't we have this in place from coast to coast? Dr. Trivedi shared her opinion: "The barrier is, say it with me, who's going to reimburse it?" Meaning, who is going to fund the training of experts and the administering of screenings and counseling and support. Not to be a Pollyanna about it, but we're discussing the psychological well-being of a significant number of people; our system needs to evaluate what we can afford.

PROVIDE CAREGIVER TRAINING AND CENTRALIZED RESOURCES

When I was introduced to the idea of administering my mom's IV medication, it freaked me out; even as I got used to it, stress was present for weeks through my paranoia that I somehow screwed up and did it wrong. More than half of Millennial caregivers assist with activities of daily living (ADLs) and/or complex medical and nursing tasks, ranging from medication management to wound care and IV administration.[9] Of the Millennials performing medical and nursing tasks, less than 28 percent received instruction (I was a lucky one, so to speak). Not to mention, research has found that caregivers who feel isolated (as many of us younger caregivers do) are at higher risk for experiencing difficulties with complex care.[10] With these experiences, it's no wonder large numbers of Millennials are skeptical of the American healthcare system; often they've been left to figure out how to perform nursing tasks on their own.[11]

As a reminder: medical or nursing tasks can include things like changing bandages on wounds or changing colostomy bags. ADLs can include helping the person you care for bathe, eat, use the bathroom, or transfer (for example, move from their wheelchair to bed or the toilet). Millennials often don't feel qualified to take on these types of tasks but don't have a choice. In addition, they're also often managing medications and dosages and monitoring the drugs' effectiveness, side effects, or changes, good or bad. Multiple caregivers told me they keep a detailed record of their family member's condition and care, logging symptoms, treatments, and results. I was my father's healthcare proxy, which meant legally I was the one to make his healthcare decisions. And while dealing with insurance companies isn't a typical medical or nursing task, it is another medical necessity we need to figure out and a huge stressor that practically every caregiver mentioned as being the bane of their existence. The time spent on hold, getting transferred and hung up on, receiving no answers. And these caregivers *needed* answers.

Even caregivers who don't assist with daily medical tasks are required to assert themselves as patient advocates, which requires a feeling of empowerment in settings that may not invite or appreciate their opinion. Caregivers of all ages report their input is at times not valued by medical professionals, even though they are the one with the best knowledge of the patient and can observe changes (in behavior, in symptoms) a stranger or someone who doesn't know the patient as well might not.

A solution: better training and resources for caregivers, for (a big) one. From the caregiver perspective, the pandemic ushered in some health-care improvements: telehealth and TeleDoc appointments not only make it possible to get the care recipient attended to more easily (don't require transportation) but also open up treatment options to those who are geo-graphically remote. But we still need resources geared toward providing the information caregivers require for at-home care that doesn't go hay-wire and leave us, as untrained caregivers, wondering if we're about to accidentally kill our loved one. This concern is real.

Who pays for caregiver training? Dr. Trivedi again shared that pay-ment is often the obstacle, though in this case the means to pay (meaning, a billing code that can be charged) exists...but is underutilized. Health-care systems need to educate themselves, she said, "because if that's the barrier, then that's available." Therapist Christina Irving described new, enhanced caregiver supports that are offered through Medicare, Medicaid, and the Older Americans Act. Their availability depends on which state you live in and your eligibility; not all caregivers are covered, but some are—a good sign of progress.

RECOGNIZE US

The medical system also needs to recognize the knowledge of caregivers and take us seriously in clinical settings. When my mom was admitted to the ER, I relayed to the emergency medicine doctor the changes I had noticed in her breathing and the sudden loss of energy and strength that my mom had attributed to "just being tired." He took me seriously. "She's her daughter," he informed another doctor. "She can tell us what's different from the norm." Considering me, and my knowledge of my mom's "typical" health baseline, helped to build my trust in him, that he was considering all sides, getting all the information, and providing her with the best care. But I've noticed through conversations with a lot of caregivers that this experience is not the norm.

One caregiver reached out to Caregiver Collective for tips on "demanding respect" in professional healthcare situations, and fellow caregivers jumped in to pep her up: *Carry yourself with authority.... Use direct eye contact.... Be fearless!* These are important bits of advice in any case, but I'd like to assert it's the medical professionals who should be taking tips from my mom's ER doctor and paying attention to family caregivers who are on the front lines daily.

Caregivers are only beginning to be recognized as an essential part of the healthcare system. When patients have family involved in their care, tangible results can be seen in their health and mortality. An article in *The Atlantic* contained a potent observation of this in patients hospitalized with COVID at the pandemic's height: doctors took note of how ICU patients improved when the doctors attempted to fill the void in comfort that a present family member would have provided.[12] Personalization, calling the patient by their name and imparting comforting words, the article noted, could mean a patient's life or death. The importance of family presence could not be questioned.

Caregivers are not just who the patient gets handed off to. There is a dire need for the medical community to recognize our true role and its necessity in positive health outcomes. Provide us with support.

CHAPTER 23

HOW *SYSTEMIC CHANGES* CAN FACILITATE NECESSARY CARE

The nature of our lives [as caregivers] can be one that is just very messy and not very cut and dry and doesn't have easy solutions to the problems that we experience. Because, in fact, a lot of the problems that we experience are systemic.... These are failures of social care nets, the healthcare nets in our system, that we are now the living embodiment of.

—Dr. Feylyn Lewis

W HEN I PROPOSE A RADICAL RETHINK TO IMPROVE THE REALITY OF care in our country, I also mean taking a look at the big picture: observing our systemic status quo and reevaluating how we've gotten used to doing things. I've touched on systemic inequities that influence caregiving and directly impact caregivers—along lines of gender, race, and economics. "Fixing" these large-scale social inequities is, for many obvious reasons, a worthwhile and necessary mission; in time, it would alleviate some of the harsh repercussions of caregiving. On a practical level, though, there are big-picture systemic changes we can make in the immediate future to improve our country's care crisis and the overall well-being of Americans.

The 2022 National Strategy to Support Family Caregivers addresses many of these, from the ability to hire affordable in-home care to redesigning Medicaid eligibility so a person or family doesn't need to deplete assets before accessing support.[1] The strategy includes 345 actions committed by fifteen agencies within the federal government to take within three years. These federal actions are all within existing programs.

"When taken as a whole," the strategy paper states, "they represent the first time that agencies across government have surveyed their own programs to identify ways of improving consistent access to supports and services for family caregivers—a significant step in and of itself."[2] Though not a be-all, end-all, the strategy includes important initiatives to address caregivers that can really help. However, while writing this book I became familiar with one overarching systemic deficiency that impacts our care and ourselves, one that needs addressing in order for provisions and programs to function well:

Our system is a disjointed mess.

We know this, right? But watching it in action (or inaction), trying to accomplish anything within it, pulls back the curtain to another level of awareness. There are supports on a federal level…statewide…or within cities, towns, and communities…but there is no cohesion or central place for information. Even federal programs like Medicaid have eligibility requirements that change from state to state. It's impossible to figure out the rules for what and where, and it's difficult to even figure out what's available to you. Without knowledge of what's out there, or a central place to begin looking and learning, a caregiver needs to figure out where to ask first, and what they're even asking for. Care support and information are completely piecemeal.

"That's the thing that is so challenging with our system, is it's not really a system," Christina Irving said. "It's just these fragmented pieces of programs that all have different eligibility, different applications." We were discussing ways in which caregivers can access support from available programs and how confusing it is even to know where to turn. "Reach out through counties, through their information and referral programs, through social workers, the hospital…If you can get connected to one community-based program, they might be able to help make links to others and understand and navigate through those, because it is hard."

Wouldn't it be helpful, instrumental even, if information on supports and resources available to you was centralized, one source? If there was a person to lessen our learning curve and walk us through the process, a seasoned professional to take our family's individual situation into account and show us how to access available programs and make care-related decisions?

Such a person, in essence, is the modern social worker in their current role, described earlier. But, in my experience and in the experiences of people I've spoken with, the social worker's work ends more or less once the person receiving care has transferred from the hospital to back home (or to in-patient rehab or a living facility). Shortly after Feylyn's mom returned home after having a stroke, the hospital social worker said, "Well, there's nothing more I can do for you." Once things seem set up for the short term, the social worker moves on. They're not at fault; that's their job and they can't continue to manage every patient they've ever helped.

But what about someone who could stay with your family through the evolution and duration of illness or disability, whom you could reach out to as needed? Someone who knows your family member's medical history, is familiar with their details, and knows how to navigate the system—from health care to benefits to community resources. A person who knows what is out there and available, which of those you are eligible for and how to apply so you are not guessing and random googling. A person who is trained to help you make the decision, "No, it's not yet time for hospice" or offer, "Yes, I can help you hire a great home aide." Imagine someone who is with you for the long haul. Can you imagine such an angel?

As we say in New York: *I gotta guy.*

CARE COORDINATORS

A care coordinator (also called a care manager) is this professional and, from what I've gathered from caregivers who have utilized their services,

they make all the difference. Care coordinators are usually social workers, psychologists, nurses, gerontologists, or others with both training
and experience in many aspects of eldercare.[3] I've heard multiple people
refer to them as the "boots on the ground." They can assess needs, handle crises (such as an emergency hospitalization), help with suggestions
and placement for long-term care facilities, mediate family disputes, identify community resources, and pinch-hit at doctor appointments when
caregivers can't make it.[4] They act as your family advocate and walk you
through decisions for which you feel in over your head. After my mom
was discharged from the hospital a few months ago, I noticed a couple
of days later that her breathing seemed heavier than normal, she looked
like she was getting weaker instead of better. I felt something was wrong,
but my mom wanted to stay home and rest. The hospital had assigned a
short-term case manager (care managers within the hospital system); not
knowing what to do, I insisted my mom call her for advice. It was the
case manager who advised me to be safe rather than sorry and to take
my mother to the emergency room right away. It was a decision that very
likely saved my mom's life.

Particularly at this life stage, when we're balancing so many things and
inexperienced with even the basics of eldercare, a care coordinator can
save us the time of reinventing the wheel and can walk us through what's
out there and how it works.

A Care Coordinator Helped Direct Lizzie Where to Go

When Lizzie's husband, who has long COVID, began experiencing symptoms, he was sent to one specialist after another and, often, they weren't
sure why. Lizzie describes it as "playing PCP [primary care physician]
whack-a-mole." The ordeal was "really frustrating" because she didn't feel
the doctors they visited cared about helping him, they just punted her
husband down the pike for another provider to figure it out. Because he
experienced fatigue, one doctor told them to see a rheumatologist. "I goo-
gled everything I could possibly find out about rheumatology. I'm like,
I don't understand why we're here," she said. With each new specialist

came the job of figuring out who to see. "We were doing it ourselves. And no one tells you a specific provider to go to, I think because they don't want to be charged with steering people. But I'm just like, 'Could you please steer us? You just hand me the whole frickin' directory and I don't know who to pick.'"

Lizzie knew she needed help she could trust. She told her husband, "'We need a quarterback of your care because it can't be me because I don't have the medical knowledge.' So we do now have a care coordinator through the long COVID program, and we have a PCP who cares and is now trying to coordinate the health stuff."

A Care Coordinator Helped Laura Hire Extra Support and Make Long-Term Decisions

When Laura's dad was dealing with the double blow of Alzheimer's and cancer, she and her brother followed advice and enlisted the help of a care coordinator, whom Laura called "a gifted person." The care coordinator had a wide network; a former nurse herself, she provided them with background information on hiring nurses and home health aides and introduced them to people she had previously worked with and recommended. I can't underscore enough how helpful this is: Kaci told me how difficult it was to find a good home aide for her mom, particularly one they could afford. Alexandra told me that even with financial resources she had a difficult time finding a home health aide for her mother; they went through official agencies, which she called "a nightmare," and after four or five aides finally landed on an aide they loved and who had the skills they needed. In contrast, Laura told me that with their care manager's help, she and her brother didn't have difficulty hiring an aide. (I'll note that, yes, they live in New York City, which is rich in resources, but just having someone recommend specific people who are already trusted is a major shortcut.)

As their dad's needs and diagnoses evolved, Laura and her brother would call the care manager periodically for guidance on how to proceed and she helped them to set it up, offering advice on round-the-clock care and whether they should opt for hospice. The care manager was already familiar with her dad, his needs, and his story; she had insight into who and what he might like and which decisions would be in line with his wishes.

How Can You Access, and Afford, a Care Coordinator?

This all sounds great, right? It also sounds expensive. If you pay out pocket, it is: a care coordinator hired privately can cost $75 to $250 per hour and isn't covered by Medicare, Medicaid, or most private insurance plans.[5] But hang on: some local organizations and government agencies offer consulting services for free or on an income-based sliding scale. Laura's family found their first care coordinator through CaringKind, a New York organization devoted to Alzheimer's caregiving that offers "caregiving coaching" free of charge.[6] Her family paid for continued use of a coordinator, but these free coaching sessions can be incredibly helpful, particularly when you're getting started.

Another hurdle that prohibits caregivers from using a care coordinator is they just don't know about this service. Lizzie knew about care coordinators because she works in health care; Laura sought one out on the advice of a family friend. Often, I recommend the use of a care coordinator to caregivers and am asked, "What's that?" It's not a widely known profession; these professionals are also not "one size fits all"; you really need someone experienced in the specific medical needs of whatever health, disability, or aging issue you are dealing with. From the benefits that I've heard from families who have utilized this type of professional guidance, it seems the experience of caregiving could be radically improved if access to this level of care coordination were a given and not a privilege for those in the know or who can afford it. No matter the care situation, use of a good care coordinator would help.

I wish I could tell you how to easily find affordable (or free) care coordinators in your area; again, the system is a disjointed mess. My best advice, as of today, is the obvious: google "care coordinators" and your state's name. You'll see pages for paid care coordinators you can hire and, hopefully, local government resources that can direct you to available programs. You can also google local organizations focused on the disease your family is dealing with, such as CaringKind. Finding a care coordinator will most likely involve digging without the promise of a holy grail outcome, which is why I bring up...

Call to Action: Universal Access to Care Coordinators

Knowing how much our country relies on caregivers to prop up the healthcare system, knowing how much more effective we would be to our economy if all caregivers (who wanted to) could actively participate in the workforce, and, most importantly, knowing how severe the personal repercussions of providing care are, shouldn't achieving universal access to this level of care assistance be a priority? Shouldn't we be putting more attention into making care coordination widely available, throughout all communities? Shouldn't we be figuring out how to have this included as a healthcare benefit?

Aha. Let's pause here for a second, because Medicare actually does offer something kinda similar. In 2015, Medicare rolled out a federal program for Chronic Care Management (CCM). To be eligible, a person must have two or more chronic conditions (at least two-thirds of Medicare enrollees do[7]) and be covered by Medicare—we're not achieving universal access with the program as is, but hell, it's a pretty solid start. The program is run typically through a PCP's office, where a qualified professional (a physician assistant or nurse practitioner) provides a consistent, non-face-to-face patient relationship. They keep records of the patient's health information and comprehensive electronic care plans, manage care transitions and other services, coordinate sharing the person's health information with specialists, engage caregivers, and help the person receiving care with preventative care and achieving health goals.[8] Often this looks like weekly phone calls to the patient, checking in on their status and medications, assessing their needs (from medical to psychosocial), and coordinating necessary community supports. Research has found the CCM program to have proven benefits, like fewer hospital visits for the patient, but "uptake has been sluggish."[9]

The problem? Many eligible medical practices refuse to implement it. In 2019, only 4 percent of eligible people participated in the CCM program, and that number seems to have held steady through 2023. NPR states:

> *Health policy experts say a host of factors limit participation in the program. Chief among them is that it requires both doctors and patients to opt in. Doctors may not have the capacity to regularly monitor patients outside office visits. Some also worry about meeting the strict Medicare documentation requirements for reimbursement and are reluctant to ask patients to join a program that may require a monthly copayment if they don't have a supplemental policy.*[10]

Some doctor offices do not want to participate because it requires extra logistics or up-front costs, like switching records to an electronic system and having a dedicated staff member fill the role. On the patient end, some people don't want to be contacted at home. From the caregiver perspective, I have to think utilizing this program would help take some stress and medical tasks off their plate. I also acknowledge that this program puts communication primarily in the hands of the person receiving care (privacy laws are a big factor), so I stand behind the use of a care coordinator to work with the family unit, but I ask this question:

If Medicare can enact the CCM program, isn't there hope that a similar program to fund care coordinators through federal benefits could be possible?

Hang on! Because just as I'm wrapping up the writing of this book, I received some good news: Medicare is launching an eight-year pilot program to assist families dealing with dementia—including a care coordinator for each family, available on-call 24/7.[11] *Chills!* The coordinator is trained in dementia care, familiar with the patient and their family, there to troubleshoot, coordinate appointments, and identify care services. The program, Guiding an Improved Dementia Experience (GUIDE), is "modeled on a handful of promising, smaller programs linked to academic institutions."[12] Patients in these programs were found to have fewer ER visits and were able to continue living at home for longer; patients in a controlled GUIDE trial program had fewer signs of dementia and their caregivers reported lower stress. "We've never tried anything like this before," said Liz Fowler, director of the Center for Medicare and Medicaid Innovation.[13]

We are on the brink of a revolution! Seriously, I am freaking out.

True, this program is only available to families dealing with dementia. True, it's an eight-year pilot program, so not yet widespread or proven—and who knows when it, or something similar, would be accessible to the many of us providing care today. But I am incredibly optimistic on how this can impact care, and its toll on us, in the future. This program could serve, hopefully, as a test run for expanded eligibility in the future.

Access to care coordinators is a solution, I believe, we would not age out of: If we could move our country in a direction in which people truly have the option of how they provide care (whether hiring affordable help, utilizing a facility, or living in themselves), a care coordinator would still be critical to help navigate illness and disability. As care access hopefully expands in the United States, this is a service that can evolve with us.

A WHITE HOUSE CAREGIVING CZAR

Whereas a care coordinator can help us individually to make sense of a fractured system, let's zoom out and consider the big picture: What can be done so the care system itself is less fractured? In a 2020 opinion piece for the *Washington Post*, Melinda Gates argued for the White House to appoint a Caregiving Czar. A czar, she wrote, is a "high-level administration role periodically created to focus accountability on key issues" (she noted that President Obama named one in 2009 to save the American auto industry). A Caregiving Czar would be a point person who could work with Congress on behalf of caregivers to pass immediate relief, "tracking policy proposals and pilot projects in cities across the country, and by encouraging innovative, market-based solutions to better serve families. Those good ideas are out there—they deserve White House attention."

> *By creating a new position to lead a multiagency caregiving response, he*
> *[the president] could ensure that, for the first time ever, the federal govern-*
> *ment is formally considering the needs of caregivers in all policy making*
> *and legislation…Because caregiving cuts across so many departments and*
> *issue areas—health, education and labor—reform is best driven by someone*
> *positioned high enough to take a sweeping view of the policy landscape and*
> *empowered with the resources and authority to elevate promising solutions.*[14]

Reading this, I'm sold. A czar could advance caregiving issues with a holistic view on caregiving across the United States, while championing and expanding local resources. The "innovative, market-based solutions" Gates references include the eldercare apps we mentioned earlier, developed by people in our generation with an eye toward caring for elders. The czar could advocate for federal laws to protect caregivers and the act of care itself, including the needs of people requiring care. A czar would not create a central system of care (truthfully, I don't think a single central system would be great: local community organizations are necessary because they have eyes and ears on the particular needs of that community; for example, accessible transportation to the doctor is not the same for someone in Chicago as it is for someone in rural Montana), but would empower a central advocate. Melinda Gates proposed this idea as a move toward gender equity, to keep women in the workforce, but knowing what we do about caregiving in our generation, I think there's a solid argument that a Caregiving Czar would have an even wider scope for positive impact.

All told, these proposals are not so radical; they are rooted in existing, proven supports that can be applied to care in new ways. The most radical element required is to change our thinking, daring to think past what is to what could be. Caregivers learn how to course correct, redrawing battle plans all the time; evolving problems require minds just as quick. It's time we take a page out of this playbook. The future of care needs to be open-minded to new possibilities, to act quickly to sustain our modern approach to this traditional role—all our health depends on it.

WHAT COMES NEXT?
OUR CONSTELLATIONS OF CARE

BEFORE I GO, THERE'S ANOTHER REPERCUSSION OF CAREGIVING I WANT to share with you:

There is something you experience after caregiving. Not during, when you are wrapped up in keeping the wheels on while simultaneously trying to make sense of what has happened in your family, what is happening to you. But on the other side, once your eyes readjust to your new surroundings: You begin to notice it *everywhere*. It's like when someone says to you, "Have you noticed how many women are pregnant lately?" And you say no, because you haven't noticed that, and then on your walk home and for the week after, all you see are pregnant women. It was brought to your attention, and now your eye quickly focuses in. That's how it is with caregiving. You notice the adult son maneuvering his mother's wheelchair through a restaurant door so they can share a nice meal together; you understand the effort that takes for both of them. You notice small acts all around you; you do them yourself for strangers because maybe you're more attuned to the needs of a person who can't get around so well or who needs help pulling that wheelchair over a curb. I remember the small acts I received, a man who rushed over to steady my dad's walker when he was effortfully lowering himself to sit on a park bench. The man was helping my dad, but, for that moment, he gave me someone to lean on, too. You begin to understand caring for others isn't only your experience; it's a truth.

I've talked about caregiving, and his illness, more since my father died, probably because the distance eases overwhelm and some pain and it's easier for me to talk about now in ways I wouldn't have allowed myself to at the time. When I think back about the experience of my dad's illness, I guess—or rightly assume—there are things I've forgotten. Feelings that, so potent at the time, probably persisted for weeks are now miles back by the wayside. I don't need them anymore. Though I focused this book on the necessary discussion of the difficulties of care and illness of someone you love, I do remember caregiving also introduced some of my most profound moments of gratitude. Days that were spent well, conversations I could still have, his gaze I could still hold—these weren't lost on me. I'd walk home elated. I also remember, really in the thick of things, looking at my mom and my dad and how strong and brave they both were and thinking: *Wow, this is the stock I come from.* It was like, by seeing their superpowers, I knew I must have superpowers too; genetically I must be strong as hell. It motivated me to keep going.

If I'm honest with myself, I wrote this book because I had to under-stand it. Not the care work per se, but us—our human condition. Our collective tug to strengthen family bonds, sometimes building them from scratch, because of or in spite of the families we were born into. In an age of such persistent divisiveness, of rampantly rewarded individualism that has initiated celebrated narcissism, I witness something different. Our desire to be a member of, to tend to, a family unit—even when it feels like our hair is on fire, even when it's the most difficult thing you've been asked to do in your life. *Of course* it's hard. We care for people because we care about them; our feelings are inextricably tied up in it. This connec-tion through care, through love, is so inherent in us, so ingrained, it gets passed on through each generation, no matter what it's named. To con-tinue caring for each other as we hope to, we need to remain mindful, to shape our present so that living our priorities is our reality, not idealism. Sometimes it's the youngest of us who see this most clearly.

Here's the thing about being a caregiver at a young age: you'll prob-ably do it again. Build your community of support. The more I witness, the more I see we have constellations of care: the people close to you in your care now may be different from the ones who support you caring for someone else later. Let yourself be pulled into someone else's constellation.

For some people, you may help by being an additional pair of boots on the ground; for others, you may call to check in. These constellations evolve, they draw new maps, they connect all of us to each other and all of us to care and to a deeper understanding of family. I look at the caregiving my mom has given to her family with new eyes.

I titled this book *Generation Care* because the more stories I heard of family illness in our generation, the clearer I saw this strong silk thread that binds us, almost invisible but obvious once you see it: it's one of care for the people of our lives, who we feel devotion to, the casual and the painstaking acts of love we exhibit daily. *Generation Care* is a testament to who we are when no one is looking, to who we continue to be.

Generation Care is also an offering to the overlooked many in our generation. A reminder of the care and comfort we deserve to receive—from ourselves and from those we casually encounter and those we hold tightly in our lives. The care and consideration we demand from institutions and bodies politic. Accepting this type of care is only a reflection of who we already are, a mirror of what we already give or gave. I hope from reading *Generation Care* that you've received some of it.

So much has happened since I began writing this book. Multiple people interviewed, who were so in the trenches when they spoke to me about the stress of their loved one's illness, have since experienced their death. Now they are the ones on the other side. Some have gotten into care advocacy work, building networks to help others; some grant themselves temporary amnesia, traveling abroad or delving back into work or the kids who still need their attention, until they are able to come to terms with what they've lived through. Some are standing still but still standing, dazed at how the hell they got there; just give them a moment to find their bearings. They've all been through a lot.

Every morning I wake up to Caregiver Collective alerts on my phone: new member requests from all over the country, new posts asking for tips on traveling with someone in a wheelchair or asking for support while they wait in a hospital hallway. In the course of my day, or my week, I talk to people about the book I'm writing and inevitably someone tells me they've lived it, too. I text with extended family and friends and hear about new diagnoses or their family member's need for an aide, and I pass along some tips, maybe something they hadn't yet thought of. I don't usually need to dig too deep in my pocket for some relevant info, but for them they are just beginning. It's been years since I was in the thick of it with my own father, feeling like I was the only one. Now the recipient of so many people's family stories, hearing what they live through and how they cope and how they hope, I am never alone.

I realize I never was.

ACKNOWLEDGMENTS

THIS BOOK IS CENTERED ON A MILLENNIAL EXPERIENCE BUT IS ULTIMATELY about family—I give big thanks to, and for, mine. I want to thank my mom, Natalie Basiuk, for supporting my writing since I was a child and now on its (often unpredictable) professional road. She didn't blink when I asked her permission to share particular family specifics in this book—and it allowed me to be most honest. Most importantly, she always supports me in the things I do or the goals I set, no matter what I've cooked up this time. I have always been loved and told I could do it.

My mom was with my father at a neurologist visit once when he was asked if he'd like to eventually donate his brain for scientific research. She was surprised when, with a resolute expression and without hesitation, he agreed. Little was known about progressive supranuclear palsy (PSP), so every opportunity to study it, to research its effects on the brain, is an important one—he was clearly proud he'd be part of that mission to find a cure. I'm confident he would feel the same about my writing this book: proud to be a part of helping others in a similar predicament, that he is definitely proud of me. I miss my father, Seth Levin, every day.

It was *Cosmopolitan* that first gave me a caregiving platform when caregiving was far from a talked-about topic among young adults. The editors there recognized it was important to speak the unspoken reality. The *Washington Post* reacted similarly when I pitched my experience with little-known caregiver PTSD—content from pages 183 and 190 of this book is drawn from that article ("I Was My Dad's Caregiver Through His Fatal Illness. I Had No Idea I'd Be at Risk for PTSD") published December 12, 2018.

Fortuitously, those articles and my (very helpful and patient) attorney, Eric Brooks, led me to my agent, Stephanie Rostan. She had listened to interviews when I had spoken on the widespread implications care has on our generation and told me, "You should be writing about *that*." It was the message and information I wanted so badly to get out there, and I feel incredibly lucky to have found the agent who heard it, recognized it (and me), and worked to amplify it.

That luck continued with Hachette Go and Balance Books. I have been writing for long enough to know what a gift it is to pair with someone who clearly sees your project's intent and potential, supports that vision (and the artistic process of the neurotic writer behind it), and provides the guardrails to keep it on track with authenticity—Renee Sedliar is that editorial shepherd. Her regular check-ins were insightful, just plain *cool*, and incredibly beneficial to the finished product—and keeping me sane. I want to thank her and the rest of the editorial team, particularly Nzinga Temu and Sean Moreau, immensely.

Many experts have answered my calls and my questions—I'd particularly like to thank C. Grace Whiting, Dr. Ranak Trivedi, Christina Irving, and Dr. Feylyn Lewis. Since we were in elementary school, Dr. Lisa Paz has provided me with mature insight well beyond her years, and including her sage expertise in this book is the cherry on top of it all.

Finally, I have such gratitude for the many people of my generation, or generation-ish, who shared with me details about their lives and their families that help to connect the dots for all of us. Opening up about illness and care can be incredibly painful, and that vulnerability requires strength; I don't take it for granted.

HELPFUL RESOURCES

<small>PLEASE NOTE: BELOW ARE RESOURCES I'VE COME ACROSS MYSELF OR</small> that have been shared among caregivers I know—they are here to get you started. Other than my own groups, Caregiver Collective and Caregiver Collective: Bulletin Board (come join us!), their inclusion should not be considered an endorsement.

GENERAL RESOURCES—GOOD STARTING POINTS

AARP's Caregiving Guide (available in English, Spanish, and Chinese)
https://www.aarp.org/caregiving/prepare-to-care-planning-guide/

Family Caregiver Services by State
https://www.caregiver.org/connecting-caregivers/services-by-state

Checklist of Documents and Legal Paperwork to Have in Order
AARP
https://www.aarp.org/caregiving/financial-legal/info-2020/caregivers-legal
-checklist.html

National Family Caregivers Association
https://nfca.typepad.com/files/checklist.pdf

Your city or state's Office for the Aging (or equivalent)

Helpful Caregiving Info, Tips, and Resources
Caregiver Collective: Bulletin Board
https://www.facebook.com/groups/caregivercollectivebulletinboard

National Council on Aging
https://www.ncoa.org/caregivers/benefits/caregiver-support/

USC Family Caregiver Support Center (even great for those not in California)
https://losangelescrc.usc.edu

CHAPTER 2: IDENTITY CRISIS AND CAREGIVING IN SILENCE

AARP Family Caregiving Guide for Asian Americans
https://www.aarp.org/content/dam/aarp/caregiving/pdf/family-caregiving
-guide/pan-asian.pdf

How to Talk to People in Your Life About Caregiving (conversation guide)
https://caringacross.org/wp-content/uploads/2024/04/CAG-Guide-For
-Caregivers.pdf

Online support group for male or Latinx caregivers caring for someone with
Alzheimer's or dementia
https://www.wearehfc.org/caregivers#ONLINE-SUPPORT-GROUPS

Peer Support: Caregiver Collective
https://www.facebook.com/groups/CaregiverCollective

CHAPTER 3: WHO WE CARE FOR

Cure PSP
https://www.psp.org

LGBTQ Community Caregiving Guide (AARP)
https://www.aarp.org/content/dam/aarp/caregiving/pdf/family-caregiving
-guide/lgbtq.pdf

"6 Questions to Ask That Will Make Caring for Older Relatives Much Easier"
(*Vox*)
https://www.vox.com/even-better/23911269/parents-caregiver-older-aging
-in-place-seniors-family-support

When Caring for a Veteran
Elizabeth Dole Foundation: Hidden Heroes
https://hiddenheroes.org

Rosalynn Carter Institute for Caregivers: Military Programs
https://rosalynncarter.org/military/

CHAPTER 4: WHERE WE LIVE AND WHO WE LIVE WITH

"Hard Topics for Planning Ahead" (HFC CareCon 2024 video)—choosing
between a multigen home or live-in facility or community
https://www.youtube.com/watch?v=Ibi37oAdnR0

"Services for Older Adults Living at Home" (National Institute on Aging)
https://www.nia.nih.gov/health/caregiving/services-older-adults-living-home

Find Care (In-Home or Living Community) Near You
Care.com

When Caregiving Long-Distance
https://www.caregiver.org/uploads/legacy/pdfs/Long_Distance_handbook.pdf

CHAPTER 5: WHY ISN'T MY SIBLING HELPING?

"Caregiving with Your Siblings" (Family Caregiver Alliance)
https://www.caregiver.org/resource/caregiving-with-your-siblings/

Caring Bridge: an app to connect and coordinate with others in your family care team
https://www.caringbridge.org

"Esther Calling: It Feels Like My Siblings Abandoned Me" (*Where Should We Begin? with Esther Perel* podcast)
https://www.estherperel.com/podcasts/esther-calling---it-feels-like-my-siblings-abandoned-me

CHAPTER 8: THE SANDWICH GENERATION GIVES RISE TO THE MULTIGENERATIONAL CAREGIVER

"Family Meeting: A Conversation with Vice President Kamala Harris" (video)
https://www.youtube.com/watch?v=IvN5JgVBSS4

CHAPTER 9: MAINTAINING FRIENDSHIPS

Simon Sinek and Trevor Noah on Friendship, Loneliness, Vulnerability, and More (video)
https://www.youtube.com/watch?v=CNBxIhxHHxM

CHAPTER 10: CAREGIVING AND OUR MENTAL HEALTH

Caregiver Crisis Textline: Rosalynn Carter Institute for Caregivers
Text TOUGH to 741741 for free, 24/7 crisis counseling

"How Can I Find Support as a Caregiver?" (Mental Health America)
https://screening.mhanational.org/content/how-can-i-find-support-caregiver/

"I Used to Be Resilient. What Happened?" (*New York Times*)
https://www.nytimes.com/2024/08/30/well/mental-resilience-tips.html

CHAPTER 11: WE'RE FEELING *ISOLATED AND ALONE*

Caregiver Collective
https://www.facebook.com/groups/CaregiverCollective

"Dr. Vivek Murthy on Loneliness and Connection" (*Unlocking Us with Brené Brown* podcast)
https://brenebrown.com/podcast/dr-vivek-murthy-and-brene-on-loneliness-and-connection/

CHAPTER 12: WE'RE FEELING *STRESSED*

"Jesus Trejo: Stay at Home Son" (comedy special)
https://tubitv.com/movies/657112/jesus-trejo-stay-at-home-son

"Mindful Meditation" (HFC CareCon 2024 video for caregivers)
https://www.youtube.com/watch?v=l-UgWNnr7qw

988 Suicide & Crisis Lifeline
Call or text 988
https://988lifeline.org

"When Caregiving Impacts Your Mental Health: 5 Tips for Talking to Your
    Employer" (Mental Health America)
https://mhanational.org/when-caregiving-impacts-your-mental-health-5-tips
    -talking-your-employer

CHAPTER 14: WE'RE FEELING *TERRIFIED AND TRAUMATIZED*

Understanding PTSD: A Guide for Family and Friends (National Center for
    PTSD)
https://www.ptsd.va.gov/publications/print/understandingptsd_family
    _booklet.pdf

VA's Caregiver Support Line
(855) 260-3274

CHAPTER 15: WE'RE FEELING *GRIEF*

"The Pandemic Helped Me Realize How Essential My Routines Are" (*New York
    Times*): How routines can help you feel a sense of control
https://www.nytimes.com/2021/04/19/health/routines-pandemic-schedules.html

"Stephen Colbert: Grateful for Grief" (*All There Is with Anderson Cooper* pod-
    cast): Meaningful listen
https://www.cnn.com/audio/podcasts/all-there-is-with-anderson-cooper
    /episodes/ae2f9ebb-1bc6-4d47-b0f0-af17008dcd0c

CHAPTER 16: WE'RE FEELING *PISSED OFF*

"Say This, Not That, When Talking to Caregivers" (AARP)
https://www.aarp.org/caregiving/life-balance/info-2019/say-this-not-that.html

CHAPTER 17: CARE VERSUS CAREER (OR, THE CAREER COMPROMISE)

Legal helpline (A Better Balance): Nonprofit legal helpline to help you under-
    stand your workplace rights when providing family care
https://www.abetterbalance.org/get-help/
1-833-NEED-ABB

Paid Family Leave Toolkit (Family Leave Workshop): How to advocate for paid
    family leave inclusive of care in your workplace
https://static1.squarespace.com/static/56018de2e4b097f984369ce2/t/5d819fbb57
    e3753573d0846c/1568776127009/Paid_Family_Leave_Toolkit_2018.pdf

"Should I Tell My Boss I'm a Caregiver?" (Workingdaughter.com)
https://workingdaughter.com/should-i-tell-my-boss-im-a-caregiver/

CHAPTER 18: WE'RE PAYING FOR IT

"Benefits Programs That Can Help Older Adults Reduce Monthly Expenses" (National Council on Aging)
https://www.ncoa.org/article/benefits-programs-that-can-help-older-adults-reduce-monthly-expenses/

Can you get paid for family care? Find out.
https://www.usa.gov/disability-caregiver

https://freedomcare.com/10-ways-to-get-paid-while-taking-care-of-a-family-member/
(not an endorsement for the company, but this webpage is a helpful resource)

"Get Paid for the Care You Provide" (AARP): Resources if you are considering whether you can get paid for family care
https://paid4care.aarpfoundation.org/

CHAPTER 19: THE CHANGES WE NEED

"Care Fellows" (Caring Across Generations)
https://caringacross.org/care-fellows/

Paid Leave for All: Get involved with national advocacy for paid family leave
https://paidleaveforall.org

"States with Workplace Laws to Help Parents and Caregivers" (AARP): Find out if your state offers paid family leave for caregiving
https://www.aarp.org/caregiving/financial-legal/info-2019/paid-family-leave-laws.html

CHAPTER 20: A BATH BOMB DOES NOT FIX THIS

"How to Find a Therapist" (*Psychology Today*): Tips/resources to find a therapist
https://www.psychologytoday.com/us/basics/therapy/how-to-find-a-therapist#how-does-one-conduct-a-phone-screen

"Maintaining Boundaries as a Caregiver: Go from Guilt to Glow" (Mental Health America): Tips for maintaining boundaries as a caregiver (I especially love no. 3: "Set boundaries according to your goals")
https://mhanational.org/maintaining-boundaries-caregiver-go-guilt-glow

"National Respite Locator Service" (National Respite Network): Caregiver respite resource
https://archrespite.org/caregiver-resources/respitelocator/

"Respite" (Elizabeth Dole Foundation Caring for Military Families): Respite programs for military caregivers
https://hiddenheroes.org/resources-online-education/respite/

"10 Best Online Therapy Services in 2024: Tried and Tested" (Forbes Health)
https://www.forbes.com/health/mind/best-online-therapy/

Managing Stress and How to Rest and Recharge
"The Seven Types of Rest That Every Person Needs" (TED)
https://ideas.ted.com/the-7-types-of-rest-that-every-person-needs/

"Rest to Success: The Seven Types of Rest You Need with Dr Saundra Dalton-Smith" (video)
https://www.youtube.com/watch?v=4F9SALVTJzI

CHAPTER 21: HOW OUR *WORKPLACE* CAN HELP US (AND THEMSELVES)

"Creating Best-in-Class Paid Leave Policies (Virtual Panel)" (Sparrow and Paid Leave US): How a company can create a best-in-class paid-leave policy for employees (webinar)
https://trysparrow.com/blog/virtual-panel-creating-best-in-class-paid-leave-policies-at-your-company/

Supporting Caregivers in the Workplace: A Practical Guide for Employers (AARP/ Northeast Business Group on Health [NEBGH])
https://nebgh.org/wp-content/uploads/2017/11/NEBGH-Caregiving_Practical-Guide-FINAL.pdf

"Working While Caring" (Rosalynn Carter Institute for Caregivers): Employer resources
https://rosalynncarter.org/working-while-caring/

CHAPTER 22: HOW THE *HEALTHCARE SYSTEM* CAN HELP US

Aging Life Care Association: Source for (paid) care coordinators
https://www.aginglifecare.org

Care Coordination (Next Step in Care): Tips on working with care coordinators
https://www.nextstepincare.org/uploads/File/Guides/Care_Coordination/Care_Coordination.pdf

"Caregiver College Video Series" (Family Caregiver Alliance): For practical tips on helping with ADLs
https://www.caregiver.org/resource/caregiver-college-video-series/

Caring for Those Who Care: Resources for Providers: Meeting the Needs of Diverse Family Caregivers (Diverse Elders Coalition): Toolkit
https://www.diverseelders.org/wp-content/uploads/2021/03/DEC-Toolkit-Final-R2.pdf

CHAPTER 23: HOW *SYSTEMIC CHANGES* CAN FACILITATE NECESSARY CARE

"Advocacy" (Rosalynn Carter Institute for Caregivers): National advocacy info
and resource
https://rosalynncarter.org/advocacy/

"Manage Your Chronic Condition" (CMS)
https://www.cms.gov/priorities/health-equity/c2c/manage-your-chronic
-condition

"What Is Chronic Care Management?" (WebMD): Understanding Medicare's
Chronic Care Management (CCM) program
https://www.webmd.com/a-to-z-guides/what-is-chronic-care-management
(Remember: access to CCM really depends on if your doctor provides it or not)

NOTES

CHAPTER 1: WHO WE ARE: A SNAPSHOT

1. Veera Korhonen, "Resident Population in the United States in 2023, by Generation," Statista, July 5, 2024, https://www.statista.com/statistics/797321/us-population-by-generation/.

2. "Memo—Millennials by the Numbers," GenForward, August 1, 2020, https://genforwardsurvey.com/2020/08/21/millennials-by-the-numbers/.

3. "Millennials: Confident. Connected. Open to Change," Pew Research Center, February 2010, https://www.pewresearch.org/wp-content/uploads/sites/20/2010/02/millennials-confident-connected-open-to-change.pdf.

4. Andrew Van Dam, "The Unluckiest Generation in U.S. History," *Washington Post*, June 5, 2020, https://www.washingtonpost.com/business/2020/05/27/millennial-recession-covid/.

5. "HHS Releases Progress Report on Federal Implementation of the National Strategy to Support Family Caregivers," US Department of Health and Human Services, September 17, 2024, https://www.hhs.gov/about/news/index.html.

6. "Long-Term Care in America: Americans Want to Age at Home," AP-NORC Center for Public Affairs Research, May 3, 2021, https://apnorc.org/projects/long-term-care-in-america-americans-want-to-age-at-home/.

7. Susan C. Reinhard, Selena Caldera, Ari Houser, and Rita Choula, "Valuing the Invaluable 2023 Update: Strengthening Supports for Family Caregivers," AARP Public Policy Institute, March 8, 2023, https://www.aarp.org/ppi/info-2015/valuing-the-invaluable-2015-update.html.

8. Lily Roberts, Mia Ives-Rublee, and Rose Khattar, "Covid-19 Likely Resulted in 1.2 Million More Disabled People by the End of 2021—Workplaces and Policy Will Need to Adapt," Center for American Progress, February 9, 2022, https://www.americanprogress.org/article/covid-19-likely-resulted-in-1-2-million-more-disabled-people-by-the-end-of-2021-workplaces-and-policy-will-need-to-adapt/; and Reinhard et al., "Valuing the Invaluable 2023 Update."

9. Reinhard et al., "Valuing the Invaluable 2023 Update."

10. Reinhard et al., "Valuing the Invaluable 2023 Update"; and "World's Older Population Grows Dramatically," National Institutes of Health, March 28, 2016, https://www.nih.gov/news-events/news-releases/worlds-older-population-grows-dramatically.

11. Deb Gordon, "60% of First-Time Caregivers Are Gen Z or Millennial, New Study Shows," *Forbes*, February 20, 2021, https://www.forbes.com/sites/debgordon/2021/02/20/60-of-first-time-caregivers-are-gen-z-or-millennial-new-study-shows/.

12. Sarah Landrum, "Millennials and the Resurgence of Emotional Intelligence," *Forbes*, April 21, 2017, https://www.forbes.com/sites/sarahlandrum/2017/04/21/millennials-and-the-resurgence-of-emotional-intelligence/.

13. Brendan Flinn, "Millennials: The Emerging Generation of Family Caregivers," AARP Public Policy Institute, May 22, 2018, https://www.aarp.org/pri/topics/ltss/family-caregiving/millennial-family-caregiving.html.

14. "The 'Typical' Millennial Caregiver," National Alliance for Caregiving and AARP, May 2020, https://www.aarp.org/content/dam/aarp/ppi/2020/05/millennial-caregiver.doi.10.26419-2Fppi.00103.013.pdf.

15. Flinn, "Millennials: The Emerging Generation."

16. Flinn, "Millennials: The Emerging Generation."

17. National Alliance for Caregiving and AARP, "The 'Typical' Millennial Caregiver."

18. Flinn, "Millennials: The Emerging Generation."

19. Reinhard et al., "Valuing the Invaluable 2023 Update."

20. Flinn, "Millennials: The Emerging Generation."

21. National Alliance for Caregiving and AARP, "The 'Typical' Millennial Caregiver."

22. Casey Leins, "Latinos, Millennials Among Groups Least Likely to Have Health Insurance," *U.S. News & World Report*, May 4, 2017, https://www.usnews.com/news/best-states/articles/2017-05-04/latinos-millennials-among-groups-least-likely-to-have-health-insurance; and Jennifer Tolbert, Patrick Drake, and Anthony Damico, "Key Facts About the Uninsured Population," KFF, December 18, 2023, https://www.kff.org/uninsured/issue-brief/key-facts-about-the-uninsured-population/.

23. Janneke van Roij, Linda Brom, Dirkje Sommeijer, Lonneke van de Poll-Franse, and Natasja Raijmakers, "Self-Care, Resilience, and Caregiver Burden in Relatives of Patients with Advanced Cancer: Results from the eQuiPe Study," *Supportive Care in Cancer* 29 (2021): 7975–7984, https://doi.org/10.1007/s00520-021-06365-9.

CHAPTER 2: IDENTITY CRISIS AND CAREGIVING IN SILENCE

1. "Caregivers in the Workplace: Finding Balance for Your Employees," New York State Office for the Aging and New York State Department of Labor, May 2022, https://aging.ny.gov/system/files/documents/2022/07/caregivers-in-workplace-guide-2022.pdf; and Lake Snell Perry & Associates, "Family Caregivers Self-Awareness and Empowerment Project: A Report on Formative Focus Groups," September 2001.

2. "A Report on Formative Focus Groups: Final Report," Family Caregivers Self-Awareness and Empowerment Project, September 2001.

3. Monica Busch, "Ai-jen Poo Explains Why We Need to Reevaluate These Harmful Caregiving Stereotypes," Bustle, January 15, 2019, https://www.bustle.com/p/ai-jen-poo-says-these-caregiving-stereotypes-are-harmful-its-time-to-reevaluate-15691540.

4. A resource for working women who also experience eldercare.

5. Marilyn M. Skaff and Leonard I. Pearlin, "Caregiving: Role Engulfment and the Loss of Self," *The Gerontologist* 32, no. 5 (October 1992): 656–664, https://doi.org/10.1093/geront/32.5.656.

6. "Survey of Self-Identified Family Caregivers," National Family Caregivers Association, 2001, https://www.caregiveraction.org/caregiver-statistics/.

7. National Family Caregivers Association, "Survey of Self-Identified Family Caregivers."

8. Flinn, "Millennials: The Emerging Generation."

9. Yanira Cruz and Ocean Le, "Why We Must Support Our Hispanic/Latinx Caregivers," *Generations Today*, July–August 2021, https://generations.asaging.org /why-we-must-support-hispaniclatinx-caregivers.

10. Reinhard et al., "Valuing the Invaluable 2023 Update."

CHAPTER 3: WHO WE CARE FOR

1. National Alliance for Caregiving and AARP, "The 'Typical' Millennial Caregiver"; and Caring Advisor, "Taking Care of Your Parents."

2. Committee on Family Caregiving for Older Adults, National Academies of Sciences, Engineering, and Medicine, "3: Family Caregiving Roles and Impacts," in *Families Caring for an Aging America*, ed. R. Schulz and J. Eden (Washington, DC: National Academies Press, 2016), https://www.ncbi.nlm.nih.gov/books/NBK396398/.

3. Rajeev Ramchand, Terri Tanielian, Michael P. Fisher, Christine Anne Vaughan, Thomas E. Trail, Caroline Batka, Phoenix Voorhies, Michael W. Robbins, Eric Robinson, and Bonnie Ghosh-Dastidar, "Hidden Heroes: America's Military Caregivers," RAND, March 31, 2014, https://www.rand.org/pubs/research_reports/RR499.html.

4. Ramchand et al., "Hidden Heroes."

5. "Caregiving in the U.S. 2020: A Focused Look at Family Caregivers of Adults Age 18 to 49," AARP and National Alliance for Caregiving, December 2020, https:// www.aarp.org/content/dam/aarp/ppi/2021/05/caregiving-in-the-united-states-18 -to-49.doi.10.26419-2Fppi.00103.023.pdf.

6. Nicole D. Ford, Douglas Slaughter, Deja Edwards, Alexandra Dalton, Cria Perrine, Anjel Vahratian, and Sharon Saydah, "Long COVID and Significant Activity Limitation Among Adults, by Age—United States, June 1–13, 2022, to June 7–19, 2023," *Morbidity and Mortality Weekly Report* 72, no. 32 (August 11, 2023): 866–870, http://dx.doi .org/10.15585/mmwr.mm7232a3.

7. "Long Covid Basics," US Centers for Disease Control and Prevention, last modified July 11, 2024, https://www.cdc.gov/covid/long-term-effects/?CDC_AAref_Val=https:// www.cdc.gov/coronavirus/2019-ncov/long-term-effects/index.html.

8. "Caregiving and Covid-19: How the Pandemic Is Expanding the Sandwich Generation," New York Life, July 7, 2024, https://www.newyorklife.com/assets/newsroom /docs/pdfs/New_York_Life_Sandwich_Gen_White_Paper.pdf.

9. Jenny Yang, "Distribution of Relationships Between Millennial Family Caregivers and Care Recipients in the U.S. in 2015," Statista, November 30, 2023, https://www.statista .com/statistics/865239/millennial-family-caregivers-and-care-recipients-relationship -in-us/.

10. Yang, "Distribution of Relationships."

11. "Family and Medical Leave Act Advisor: Reasons for Leave—Family Member's Serious Health Condition," US Department of Labor, https://webapps.dol.gov/elaws /whd/fmla/10b1.aspx#:~:text=The%20FMLA%20allows%20leave%20for,standing %20"in%20loco%20parentis".

Chapter 4: Where We Live and Who We Live With

1. Richard Fry, Jeffrey S. Passel, and D'Vera Cohn, "A Majority of Young Adults in the U.S. Live with Their Parents for the First Time Since the Great Depression," Pew Research Center, September 4, 2020, https://www.pewresearch.org/short-reads/2020/09/04/a-majority-of-young-adults-in-the-u-s-live-with-their-parents-for-the-first-time-since-the-great-depression/.

2. Treh Manhertz, "Almost 3 Million Adults Moved Back Home in Wake of Coronavirus," Zillow, June 10, 2020, https://www.zillow.com/research/coronavirus-adults-moving-home-27271/.

3. D'Vera Cohn and Jeffrey S. Passel, "A Record 64 Million Americans Live in Multigenerational Households," Pew Research Center, April 5, 2018, https://www.pewresearch.org/short-reads/2018/04/05/a-record-64-million-americans-live-in-multigenerational-households/.

4. Kristen Bialik and Richard Fry, "Millennial Life: How Young Adulthood Today Compares with Prior Generations," Pew Research Center, February 14, 2019, https://www.pewresearch.org/social-trends/2019/02/14/millennial-life-how-young-adulthood-today-compares-with-prior-generations-2/.

5. Manhertz, "Almost 3 Million Adults Moved Back Home."

6. "Our Life Was Languid," opinion, *New York Times*, July 17, 2020, https://www.nytimes.com/2020/07/17/opinion/coronavirus-family.html.

7. William H. Frey, "The U.S. Will Become 'Minority White' in 2045, Census Projects," Brookings Institution, September 10, 2018, https://www.brookings.edu/articles/the-us-will-become-minority-white-in-2045-census-projects/.

8. Anna Wilde Mathews and Tom McGinty, "Covid Spurs Families to Shun Nursing Homes, a Shift That Appears Long Lasting," *Wall Street Journal*, December 21, 2020, https://www.wsj.com/articles/covid-spurs-families-to-shun-nursing-homes-a-shift-that-appears-long-lasting-11608565170#:~:text=The%20U.S.%20has%20the%20largest,long%2Dterm%2Dcare%20institutions.

9. "New Report Finds Access to Nursing Home Care a Growing Crisis," American Health Care Association, August 23, 2023, https://www.ahcancal.org/News-and-Communications/Press-Releases/Pages/New-Report-Finds-Access-To-Nursing-Home-Care-A-Growing-Crisis-.aspx.

10. Emmie Martin, "59% of Millennials in the U.S. Would Move to Another Country for a Job," *Business Insider*, October 7, 2014, https://www.businessinsider.com/millennials-moving-abroad-for-jobs-2014-10.

11. Caring Advisor, "Taking Care of Your Parents."

12. Caring Advisor, "Taking Care of Your Parents."

13. Caring Advisor, "Taking Care of Your Parents."

14. William A. Vega, María P. Aranda, and Francisca S. Rodriguez, "Millennials and Dementia Caregiving in the United States," Youth Against Alzheimer's, USC Suzanne Dworak-Peck School of Social Work, USC Edward R. Roybal Institute on Aging, 2017, https://www.usagainstalzheimers.org/sites/default/files/Dementia%20Caregiver%20Report_Final.pdf.

15. Committee on Family Caregiving for Older Adults, "3: Family Caregiving Roles and Impacts."

16. Mathews and McGinty, "Covid Spurs Families to Shun Nursing Homes."

CHAPTER 5: WHY ISN'T MY SIBLING HELPING?

1. Jody Gastfriend, "When Siblings Share the Caregiving for an Aging Parent, Will It Be Welfare or Warfare?" *Forbes*, August 29, 2018, https://www.forbes.com/sites /jodygastfriend/2018/08/29/15siblings-caring-for-parents/.

2. Mark É. Czeisler, Elizabeth A. Rohan, Stephanie Melillo, Jennifer L. Matjasko, Lara DePadilla, Chirag G. Patel, Matthew D. Weaver et al., "Mental Health Among Parents of Children Aged <18 Years and Unpaid Caregivers of Adults During the COVID-19 Pandemic—United States, December 2020 and February–March 2021," *Morbidity and Mortality Weekly Report* 70, no. 24 (June 18, 2021): 879–887, http://dx.doi.org/10.15585 /mmwr.mm7024a3.

CHAPTER 6: ROMANTIC RELATIONSHIPS ARE HARD AND WILL I GET TO HAVE KIDS?

1. Bialik and Fry, "Millennial Life: How Young Adulthood Today."

2. Amanda Barroso, Kim Parker, and Jesse Bennett, "As Millennials Near 40, They're Approaching Family Life Differently Than Previous Generations," Pew Research Center, May 27, 2020, https://www.pewresearch.org/social-trends/2020/05/27/as-millennials -near-40-theyre-approaching-family-life-differently-than-previous-generations/.

3. Barroso, Parker, and Bennett, "As Millennials Near 40."

4. Gretchen Livingston, "They're Waiting Longer, but U.S. Women Today More Likely to Have Children Than a Decade Ago," Pew Research Center, January 18, 2018, https://www.pewresearch.org/social-trends/2018/01/18/theyre-waiting-longer-but-u-s -women-today-more-likely-to-have-children-than-a-decade-ago/.

5. Caring Advisor, "Taking Care of Your Parents."

6. Caring Advisor, "Taking Care of Your Parents."

7. Caring Advisor, "Taking Care of Your Parents."

8. Caring Advisor, "Taking Care of Your Parents."

9. "The Only-Child Family," *Psychology Today*, July 9, 2024, https://www.psychology today.com/ie/basics/family-dynamics/only-child-family.

10. Caitlin Gibson, "The Rise of the Only Child: How America Is Coming Around to the Idea of 'Just One,'" *Washington Post*, June 19, 2019, https://www.washingtonpost.com /lifestyle/on-parenting/the-rise-of-the-only-child-how-america-is-coming-around-to -the-idea-of-just-one/2019/06/19/b4f75480-8eb9-11e9-8f69-a2795fca3343_story.html.

11. "LGBTQ Family Building Survey," Family Equity, 2019, https://www.family equality.org/resources/lgbtq-family-building-survey/.

12. Martha J. Bailey, Janet Currie, and Hannes Schwandt, "The Covid-19 Baby Bump: The Unexpected Increase in U.S. Fertility Rates in Response to the Pandemic," National Bureau of Economic Research, Working Paper No. 30569, October 2022, revised August 2023, https://www.nber.org/system/files/working_papers/w30569/w30 569.pdf.

13. Laura St. James, "The Modern Family," *Vox*, November 25, 2021, https://www.vox .com/the-highlight/22784054/estrangement-family-friends-friendsgiving.

14. Christopher Cameron, "Seven Chinese Girlfriends Buy Mansion to Retire and Die Together," *New York Post*, July 3, 2019, https://nypost.com/2019/07/03/seven -chinese-girlfriends-buy-mansion-to-retire-and-die-together/.

CHAPTER 8: THE SANDWICH GENERATION GIVES RISE TO THE MULTIGENERATIONAL CAREGIVER

1. Sarah E. Patterson and Rachel Margolis, "The Demography of Multigenerational Caregiving: A Critical Aspect of the Gendered Life Course," *Socius*, July 25, 2019, https:// doi.org/10.1177/2378023119862737.

2. New York Life, "Caregiving and Covid-19."

3. Barroso, Parker, and Bennett, "As Millennials Near 40."

4. Patterson and Margolis, "The Demography of Multigenerational Caregiving."

5. Patterson and Margolis, "The Demography of Multigenerational Caregiving."

6. New York Life, "Caregiving and Covid-19."

7. Jeff From, "Creating Meaningful Moments for Millennial Families," *Forbes*, June 26, 2018, https://www.forbes.com/sites/jefffromm/2018/06/19/creating-meaningful -moments-for-millennial-families/.

CHAPTER 10: CAREGIVING AND OUR MENTAL HEALTH

1. Scott Barry Kaufman, "Post-traumatic Growth: Finding Meaning and Creativity in Adversity," *Scientific American*, April 20, 2020, https://blogs.scientificamerican.com /beautiful-minds/post-traumatic-growth-finding-meaning-and-creativity-in-adversity/.

2. Pooja, Nitesh Bhatia, and Pranab Kumar, "Emotional Intelligence Amongst Mil- lennials: Male vs. Female Leaders in the IT and ITES Sectors," *International Journal of Human Capital and Information Technology Professionals* 13, no. 1 (2022): 1–18, http:// doi.org/10.4018/IJHCITP.300316.

3. "The Economic Consequences of Millennial Health," Moody's Analytics and Blue Cross Blue Shield, November 6, 2019, https://www.bcbs.com/sites/default/files/file -attachments/health-of-america-report/HOA-Moodys-Millennial-10-30.pdf.

4. Olga Khazan, "The Millennial Mental-Health Crisis," *The Atlantic*, June 11, 2020, https://www.theatlantic.com/health/archive/2020/06/why-suicide-rates-among -millennials-are-rising/612943/.

5. "Millennials Are 'Canaries in the Coalmine' for Toxic Economic Trends, Say Stanford Scholars," Stanford University, June 6, 2019, https://news.stanford.edu/stories /2019/06/toxic-economic-trends-impacted-millennials.

6. Khazan, "The Millennial Mental-Health Crisis."

7. Khazan, "The Millennial Mental-Health Crisis."

8. Czeisler et al., "Mental Health Among Parents of Children."

9. Kaitlin Grelle, Neha Shrestha, Megan Ximenes, Jessica Perrotte, Millie Cordaro, Rebecca G. Deason, and Krista Howard, "The Generation Gap Revisited: Generational Differences in Mental Health, Maladaptive Coping Behaviors, and Pandemic-Related

Concerns During the Initial COVID-19 Pandemic," *Journal of Adult Development*, February 16, 2023, https://www.ncbi.nlm.nih.gov/pmc/articles/PMC9934502/.

10. Eilene Zimmerman, "What Makes Some People More Resilient Than Others," *New York Times*, June 21, 2020, https://www.nytimes.com/2020/06/18/health/resilience-relationships-trauma.html.

11. Czeisler et al., "Mental Health Among Parents of Children."

12. Czeisler et al., "Mental Health Among Parents of Children."

13. Czeisler et al., "Mental Health Among Parents of Children."

14. Czeisler et al., "Mental Health Among Parents of Children."

15. Erica Coe, Jenny Cordina, Kana Enomoto, Raelyn Jacobson, Sharon Mei, and Nikhil Seshan, "Addressing the Unprecedented Behavioral-Health Challenges Facing Generation Z," McKinsey & Company, January 14, 2022, https://www.mckinsey.com/industries/healthcare/our-insights/addressing-the-unprecedented-behavioral-health-challenges-facing-generation-z.

16. Christianna Silva, "The Millennial Obsession with Self-Care," NPR, June 4, 2017, https://www.npr.org/2017/06/04/531051473/the-millennial-obsession-with-self-care.

17. Jenny Marie, "Millennials and Mental Health," National Alliance on Mental Illness, February 27, 2019, https://www.nami.org/family-member-caregivers/millennials-and-mental-health/.

18. Kaufman, "Post-traumatic Growth."

CHAPTER 11: WE'RE FEELING *ISOLATED AND ALONE*

1. Anna Gotlib, "Letting Go of Familiar Narratives as Tragic Optimism in the Era of COVID-19," *Journal of Medical Humanities* 42, no. 1 (2021): 81–101, https://doi.org/10.1007/s10912-021-09680-8.

2. Jamie Ballard, "Millennials Are the Loneliest Generation," YouGov, July 30, 2019, https://today.yougov.com/topics/society/articles-reports/2019/07/30/loneliness-friendship-new-friends-poll-survey.

3. Christopher Bergland, "Social Media Exacerbates Perceived Isolation," *Psychology Today*, March 7, 2017, https://www.psychologytoday.com/us/blog/the-athletes-way/201703/social-media-exacerbates-perceived-social-isolation.

4. Noam Shpancer, "Face-to-Face Communication: Healthier Than Digital?" *Psychology Today*, May 30, 2023, https://www.psychologytoday.com/intl/blog/insight-therapy/202305/face-to-face-communication-healthier-than-digital.

5. Richard Weissbourd, Milena Batanova, Virginia Lovison, and Eric Torres, "Loneliness in America: How the Pandemic Has Deepened an Epidemic of Loneliness and What We Can Do About It," Harvard Graduate School of Education and Making Caring Common Project, February 2021, https://mcc.gse.harvard.edu/reports/loneliness-in-america.

6. Vivek H. Murthy, "Surgeon General: We Have Become a Lonely Nation, It's Time to Fix That," *New York Times*, April 30, 2023, https://www.nytimes.com/2023/04/30/opinion/loneliness-epidemic-america.html.

7. National Alliance for Caregiving and AARP, "The 'Typical' Millennial Caregiver."

8. Bergland, "Social Media."

9. Murthy, "We Have Become a Lonely Nation."

Chapter 12: We're Feeling *Stressed*

1. "Younger Adults' Experiences and Views on Long-Term Care," AP-NORC Center for Public Affairs Research, 2018, https://apnorc.org/projects/younger-adults -experiences-and-views-on-long-term-care/.

2. "Burnout: Symptoms and Signs," WebMD, March 5, 2024, https://www.webmd.com /mental-health/burnout-symptoms-signs.

3. Morgan Smith, "Burnout Is on the Rise Worldwide—and Gen Z, Young Millennials and Women Are the Most Stressed," Make It, CNBC, March 14, 2023, https://www .cnbc.com/2023/03/14/burnout-is-on-the-rise-gen-z-millennials-and-women-are-the -most-stressed.html.

4. "Perfectionism Among Young People Significantly Increased Since 1980s, Study Finds," press release, American Psychological Association, 2018, https://www.apa.org /news/press/releases/2018/01/perfectionism-young-people.

5. Megan C. Thomas Hebdon, Miranda Jones, Sara Neller, Jacqueline Kent-Marvick, Michael Thomas, Elina Stewart, Siobhan Aaron, Christina Wilson, Neil Peterson, and Lee Ellington, "Stress and Supportive Care Needs of Millennial Caregivers: A Qualitative Analysis," *Western Journal of Nursing Research* 44, no. 3 (2022): 205–213, https://doi .org/10.1177/01939459211056689.

6. Vivian C. McAlister, "Caregiver Fatigue and Surrogate End-of-Life Decision Making," *Canadian Journal of Surgery* 59, no. 2 (2016): 77–78, https://doi.org/10.1503/cjs .002616.

7. Hebdon et al., "Stress and Supportive Care Needs."

8. "Adjustment Disorders," Mayo Clinic, July 9, 2024, https://www.mayoclinic.org /diseases-conditions/adjustment-disorders/symptoms-causes/syc-20355224.

9. "The Impact of Caregiving on Mental and Physical Health," Blue Cross Blue Shield, September 9, 2020, https://www.bcbs.com/news-and-insights/report/the-impact -of-caregiving-on-mental-and-physical-health.

10. Hebdon et al., "Stress and Supportive Care Needs."

11. Hebdon et al., "Stress and Supportive Care Needs."

12. "Caregiver Burnout," Cleveland Clinic, July 9, 2024, https://my.clevelandclinic .org/health/diseases/9225-caregiver-burnout.

13. Cleveland Clinic, "Caregiver Burnout."

14. McAlister, "Caregiver Fatigue."

15. Sara Berg, "What Doctors Wish Patients Knew About Decision Fatigue," American Medical Association, November 19, 2021, https://www.ama-assn.org/delivering -care/public-health/what-doctors-wish-patients-knew-about-decision-fatigue.

16. Pamela Rosenblum, "Decision Fatigue, 'The Numbness You Feel at the End of an Overloaded Day,'" Lewy Body Dementia Resource Center, February 22, 2022, https:// lewybodyresourcecenter.org/decision-fatigue-the-numbness-you-feel-at-the-end -of-an-overloaded-day/.

17. Rosenblum, "Decision Fatigue."

18. Danielle Page, "Caregiver Decision Fatigue: How to Know If You're Suffering from It and Ways to Cope," Care.com, September 1, 2022, https://www.care.com/c/caregiver-decision-fatigue/.

19. AARP and National Alliance for Caregiving, "Caregiving in the U.S. 2020."

20. Blue Cross Blue Shield, "The Impact of Caregiving."

21. Hebdon et al., "Stress and Supportive Care Needs."

22. Hannes Schwandt and Till M. von Wachter, "Life-Cycle Impacts of Graduating in a Recession," *The Reporter*, National Bureau of Economic Research, March 31, 2023, https://www.nber.org/reporter/2023number1/life-cycle-impacts-graduating-recession.

23. AARP and National Alliance for Caregiving, "Caregiving in the U.S. 2020."

CHAPTER 13: WE'RE FEELING *GUILTY*

1. Brittany Wong, "The 6 Things Millennials Bring Up the Most in Therapy," *HuffPost*, September 5, 2019, https://www.huffpost.com/entry/millennial-therapy-issues_n_5a0620f2e4b01d21c83e84d2.

2. "Which Generation Struggles to Set Boundaries the Most?" blog, Thriving Center of Psych, October 28, 2022, https://thrivingcenterofpsych.com/blog/setting-healthy-boundaries/.

3. Thriving Center of Psych, "Which Generation Struggles to Set Boundaries the Most?"

4. Ozlem Koseoglu Ornek and Nurcan Kolac, "Quality of Life in Employee with Workaholism," in *Occupational Wellbeing*, ed. Kanitha Palaniappan and Pamela McCauley (Open access, August 2021), https://doi.org/10.5772/intechopen.95353.

5. Anne Helen Petersen, "How Millennials Became the Burnout Generation," BuzzFeed News, January 5, 2019, https://www.buzzfeednews.com/article/annehelenpetersen/millennials-burnout-generation-debt-work; and Sarah Green Carmichael, "Millennials Are Actually Workaholics, According to Research," *Harvard Business Review*, August 17, 2016, https://hbr.org/2016/08/millennials-are-actually-workaholics-according-to-research.

6. Pete Syme, "Millennials Cared Little for Work-Life Balance But Now Changed," *Business Insider*, September 2023, https://www.businessinsider.com/millennials-cared-little-for-work-life-balance-but-now-changed-2023-9.

7. Kendall Green and Michael Stallone, "What Millennials Are Doing to Confront the 'Quarter-Life Crisis,'" Fox5 New York, April 26, 2024, https://www.fox5ny.com/news/quarter-life-crisis-marathon-running.

8. Thriving Center of Psych, "Which Generation Struggles to Set Boundaries the Most?"

9. Haley Yamada, "'Bare Minimum Mondays' Trend Sees Young Workers Setting Boundaries," ABC News, April 10, 2023, https://abcnews.go.com/GMA/Living/bare-minimum-mondays-work-trend-sheds-light-care/story?id=98464163.

CHAPTER 14: WE'RE FEELING *TERRIFIED AND TRAUMATIZED*

1. "Acute Stress Disorder," PTSD: National Center for PTSD, US Department of Veterans Affairs, July 9, 2024, https://www.ptsd.va.gov/understand/related/acute_stress.asp.

2. "What Is Posttraumatic Stress Disorder (PTSD)?" American Psychiatric Association, July 9, 2024, https://www.psychiatry.org/patients-families/ptsd/what-is-ptsd.

3. Amy B. Petrinec and Barbara J. Daly, "Post-traumatic Stress Symptoms in Post-ICU Family Members: Review and Methodological Challenges," *Western Journal of Nursing Research* 38, no. 1 (January 2016): 57–78, https://doi.org/10.1177/0193945914544176; Wendy G. Anderson, Robert M. Arnold, Derek C. Angus, and Cindy L. Bryce, "Post-traumatic Stress and Complicated Grief in Family Members of Patients in the Intensive Care Unit," *Journal of General Internal Medicine* 23, no. 11 (November 2008): 1871–1876, https://doi.org/10.1007/s11606-008-0770-2; and Jennifer L. McAdam, Dorrie K. Fontaine, Douglas B. White, Kathleen A. Dracup, and Kathleen A. Puntillo, "Psychological Symptoms of Family Members of High-Risk Intensive Care Unit Patients," *American Journal of Critical Care* 21, no. 6 (November 2012): 386–393, https://doi.org/10.4037/ajcc2012582.

4. Ronald L. Hickman Jr. and Sara L. Douglas, "Impact of Chronic Critical Illness on the Psychological Outcomes of Family Members," *AACN Advanced Critical Care* 21, no. 1 (January–March 2010): 80–91, https://doi.org/10.1097/NCI.0b013e3181c930a3.

5. Hickman and Douglas, "Impact of Chronic Critical Illness."

6. Karmel W. Choi, Kelly M. Shaffer, Emily L. Zale, Christopher J. Funes, Karestan C. Koenen, Tara Tehan, Jonathan Rosand, and Ana-Maria Vranceanu, "Early Risk and Resiliency Factors Predict Chronic Posttraumatic Stress Disorder in Caregivers of Patients Admitted to a Neuroscience ICU," *Critical Care Medicine* 46, no. 5 (May 2018): 713–719, https://doi.org/10.1097/CCM.0000000000002988.

7. Christine Sanderson, Elizabeth A. Lobb, Jane Mowll, Phyllis N. Butow, Naomi McGowan, and Melanie A. Price, "Signs of Post-traumatic Stress Disorder in Caregivers Following an Expected Death: A Qualitative Study," *Palliative Medicine* 27, no. 7 (July 2013): 625–631, https://doi.org/10.1177/0269216313483663.

8. Janet M. Cromer, "After Brain Injury: Post-traumatic Stress Grips Caregivers," *Psychology Today*, November 29, 2012, https://www.psychologytoday.com/us/blog/professor-cromer-learns-read/201211/after-brain-injury-post-traumatic-stress-grips-caregivers.

9. Cromer, "After Brain Injury."

10. Rachel Dekel and Candice M. Monson, "Military-Related Post-traumatic Stress Disorder and Family Relations: Current Knowledge and Future Directions," *Aggression and Violent Behavior* 15, no. 4 (July–August 2010): 303–309, https://doi.org/10.1016/j.avb.2010.03.001.

11. "The Secondary Trauma of PTSD in Veteran Families and Caregivers," Wounded Warrior Project, July 9, 2024, https://newsroom.woundedwarriorproject.org/A-Family-Affair-The-Secondary-Trauma-of-PTSD.

12. Claudia Carmassi, Claudia Foghi, Valerio Dell'Oste, Carlo Antonio Bertelloni, Andrea Fiorillo, and Liliana Dell'Osso, "Risk and Protective Factors for PTSD in Caregivers of Adult Patients with Severe Medical Illnesses: A Systematic Review," *International Journal of Environmental Research and Public Health* 17, no. 16 (2020): 5888, https://doi.org/10.3390/ijerph17165888.

13. Ask Elklit, Nina Reinholt, Louise H. Nielsen, Alon Blum, Mathias Lasgaard, "Post-traumatic Stress Disorder Among Bereaved Relatives of Cancer Patients," *Journal of*

Psychosocial Oncology 28, no. 4 (2010): 399–412, https://doi.org/10.1080/07347332.2010 .488142; and Richard Schulz and Paula R. Sherwood, "Physical and Mental Health Effects of Family Caregiving," *American Journal of Nursing* 108, no. 9 (Suppl. 2008): 23–27, https://doi.org/10.1097/01.NAJ.0000336406.45248.4c.

14. "Complex Post-traumatic Stress Disorder (Complex PTSD)," Medical News Today, July 9, 2024, https://www.medicalnewstoday.com/articles/322886.

15. Carmassi et al., "Risk and Protective Factors for PTSD."

16. "Acute Stress Disorder," Cleveland Clinic, February 21, 2023, https://my.cleveland clinic.org/health/diseases/24755-acute-stress-disorder.

17. "Taking Care of YOU: Self-Care for Family Caregivers," Family Caregiver Alliance, https://www.caregiver.org/taking-care-you-self-care-family-caregivers.

CHAPTER 15: WE'RE FEELING *GRIEF*

1. Einat Yehene, Alexander Manevich, and Simon Shimshon Rubin, "Caregivers' Grief in Acquired Non-death Interpersonal Loss (NoDIL): A Process Based Model with Implications for Theory, Research, and Intervention," *Frontiers in Psychology* 12 (April 2021): 676536, https://doi.org/10.3389/fpsyg.2021.676536.

2. Yehene, Manevich, and Rubin, "Caregivers' Grief."

3. Yehene, Manevich, and Rubin, "Caregivers' Grief."

4. Neerjah Skantharajah, Carol Barrie, Sharon Baxter, M. Carolina Borja, Anica Butters, Deborah Dudgeon, Ayeshah Haque et al., "The Grief and Bereavement Experiences of Informal Caregivers: A Scoping Review of the North American Literature," *Journal of Palliative Care* 37, no. 2 (2022): 242–258, https://doi.org/10.1177/08258597211052269.

5. Lauren Stroshane, "Ambiguous Loss and Anticipatory Grief—Webinar Notes," Stanford PD Community Blog, Stanford Medicine, April 20, 2020, https://parkinsons blog.stanford.edu/2020/04/ambiguous-loss-and-anticipatory-grief-webinar-notes/.

6. "Anticipatory Grief and Ambiguous Loss," Stanford Parkinson's Community Outreach, Stanford Medicine, August 2020, https://med.stanford.edu/parkinsons /caregiver-corner/caregiving-topics/anticipatory-grief.html.

7. Yehene, Manevich, and Rubin, "Caregivers' Grief."

8. "How to Handle Ambiguous Loss as a Caregiver," blog, California Caregiver Resource Centers, https://www.caregivercalifornia.org/2021/12/27/how-to-handle -ambiguous-loss-as-a-caregiver/.

9. Yehene, Manevich, and Rubin, "Caregivers' Grief."

10. "Caregiving, Grieving and Loss," fact sheet, Parkinson Canada, https:// parkinsonca.thedev.ca/wp-content/uploads/Caregiving-Grieving.pdf.

11. Stanford Medicine, "Anticipatory Grief and Ambiguous Loss."

12. Parkinson Canada, "Caregiving, Grieving and Loss."

13. Parkinson Canada, "Caregiving, Grieving and Loss."

14. "Recognizing and Coping with Anticipatory Grief," Caregiver Training Blog, mmLearn.org, October 15, 2021, https://training.mmlearn.org/blog/recognizing-and -coping-with-anticipatory-grief.

15. PDQ Supportive and Palliative Care Editorial Board, "Grief, Bereavement, and Loss (PDQ): Patient Version," in *PDQ Cancer Information Summaries* (Bethesda, MD: National Cancer Institute, 2021), https://www.ncbi.nlm.nih.gov/books/NBK65826/.

16. PDQ Supportive and Palliative Care Editorial Board, "Grief, Bereavement, and Loss."

17. Kathrin Boerner, Richard Schulz, and Amy Horowitz, "Positive Aspects of Caregiving and Adaptation to Bereavement," *Psychology and Aging* 19, no. 4 (2004): 668–675, https://doi.org/10.1037/0882-7974.19.4.668.

CHAPTER 16: WE'RE FEELING *PISSED OFF*

1. Debbie M., "Caregivers Are Over Your Toxic Positivity," Medium, March 15, 2021, https://debbiemaley.medium.com/caregivers-are-over-your-toxic-positivity -7b79f56153fa.

CHAPTER 17: CARE VERSUS CAREER (OR, THE CAREER COMPROMISE)

1. Frank Witsil and Zlati Meyer, "Millennials Aim to Attain American Dream, but Can They?" *Detroit Free Press*, June 14, 2016, https://eu.freep.com/story/money /business/2016/06/14/millennials-american-dream-economy-detroit/85559382/.

2. Dee Gill, "Entering the Job Market in Recession: The Prognosis Worsens," *UCLA Anderson Review*, April 8, 2020, https://anderson-review.ucla.edu/recession-graduate/.

3. "The Career Effects of Graduating in a Recession," National Bureau of Economic Research, November 1, 2006, https://www.nber.org/digest/nov06/career -effects-graduating-recession; Hannes Schwandt and Till M. von Wachter, "Life-Cycle Impacts of Graduating in a Recession," *The Reporter*, National Bureau of Economic Research, March 31, 2023, https://www.nber.org/reporter/2023number1 /life-cycle-impacts-graduating-recession.

4. Amy Adkins, "Millennials: The Job-Hopping Generation," Gallup, https://www .gallup.com/workplace/231587/millennials-job-hopping-generation.aspx.

5. Brad Harrington, Fred Van Deusen, Jennifer Sabatini Fraone, and Jeremiah Moerlock, "How Millennials Navigate Their Careers: Young Adult Views on Work, Life and Success," Boston College Center for Work and Family, 2015, https://www.bc .edu/content/dam/files/centers/cwf/research/publications/researchreports/how -millennials-navigate-their-careers.pdf.

6. Flinn, "Millennials: The Emerging Generation."

7. Flinn, "Millennials: The Emerging Generation."

8. National Bureau of Economic Research, "The Career Effects of Graduating in a Recession."

9. Flinn, "Millennials: The Emerging Generation."

10. Flinn, "Millennials: The Emerging Generation."

11. Ruth Reader, "Harvard Study: Workers Are Facing a Caregiving Crisis and Companies Refuse to Acknowledge It," *Fast Company*, January 16, 2019, https://www .fastcompany.com/90292935/harvard-study-workers-are-facing-a-caregiving-crisis and-companies-refuse-to-acknowledge-it.

12. Rakesh Kochhar, "Hispanic Women, Immigrants, Young Adults, Those with Less Education Hit Hardest by COVID-19 Job Losses," Pew Research Center, June 9, 2020, https://www.pewresearch.org/short-reads/2020/06/09/hispanic-women-immigrants -young-adults-those-with-less-education-hit-hardest-by-covid-19-job-losses/.

13. Wikipedia, s.v. "Family responsibilities discrimination in the United States," last modified November 4, 2023, https://en.wikipedia.org/wiki/Family_responsibilities _discrimination_in_the_United_States.

14. Reader, "Harvard Study."

15. "Family Caregivers: Information on the Family and Medical Leave Act," Wage and Hour Division, US Department of Labor, https://www.dol.gov/agencies/whd /fmla/family-caregiver.

16. "Paid Family Leave Across OECD Countries," Bipartisan Policy Center, updated September 2022, https://bipartisanpolicy.org/explainer/paid-family -leave-across-oecd-countries/#:~:text=Last%20updated%20September%202022.,ing %20or%20medical%20leave%20policy.

17. "Hilarity for Charity: Lauren Miller Rogen's Big Idea That Might Change the World," *Authority Magazine*, Medium, April 21, 2023, https://medium.com/authority -magazine/hilarity-for-charity-lauren-miller-rogens-big-idea-that-might-change -the-world-172b1588a3fd.

CHAPTER 18: WE'RE PAYING FOR IT

1. Reid Cramer, Fenaba R. Addo, Colleen Campbell, Jung Choi, Brent J. Cohen, Cathy Cohen, William R. Emmons et al., "The Emerging Millennial Wealth Gap: Divergent Trajectories, Weak Balance Sheets, and Implications for Social Policy," New America, October 29, 2019, https://www.newamerica.org/millennials/reports /emerging-millennial-wealth-gap/.

2. Cramer et al., "The Emerging Millennial Wealth Gap."

3. Cramer et al., "The Emerging Millennial Wealth Gap." This study noted the average wealth holdings for a Black Millennial were more than four times less than for a white Millennial; Hispanic Millennials sat in between.

4. Dr. Feylyn Lewis also mentioned ways in which generational wealth (particularly in light of race) can affect the ways we care and the options we have when it comes to private pay or external resources. For example, did we grow up with hired caregivers in our family, or was taking on our own family care always the norm? Were we raised in a resource-rich area, or is our family's district more strapped? Do we pay for more out-of-pocket care expenses than our more affluent peers whose family can afford care themselves?

5. Hanneh Bareham, "Which Generation Has the Most Student Loan Debt?" Bankrate, September 28, 2023, https://www.bankrate.com/loans/student-loans /student-loan-debt-by-generation/#stats.

6. Minda Zetlin, "63 Percent of Millennials Have More Than $10,000 in Student Debt. They'll Be Paying for Decades," *Inc.*, January 11, 2017, https://www.inc.com /minda-zetlin/63-percent-of-millennials-have-more-than-10000-in-student-debt-theyll -be-paying.html.

7. Shelly Banjo, "A Decade's Worth of Progress for Working Women Evaporated Overnight," Bloomberg, June 3, 2020, https://www.bloomberg.com/news/articles/2020 -06-03/coronavirus-is-disproportionately-impacting-women.

8. Banjo, "A Decade's Worth of Progress."

9. New York Life, "Caregiving and COVID-19."

10. Tom Risen, "1 in 4 Americans Lack Emergency Savings," *U.S. News & World Report*, June 23, 2014, https://www.usnews.com/news/blogs/data-mine/2014/06/23/1-in-4-americans-lack-emergency-savings.

11. Sarah Foster, "Survey: More Than Half of Americans Couldn't Cover Three Months of Expenses with an Emergency Fund," Bankrate, July 21, 2021, https://www.bankrate.com/banking/savings/emergency-savings-survey-july-2021/.

12. New York Life, "Caregiving and COVID-19."

13. Laura Alpert, "Frugality Comeback: Many Millennials Thriftier Than Other Generations," *The Ledger*, May 29, 2013, https://eu.theledger.com/story/news/2013/05/29/frugality-comeback-many-millennials-thriftier-than-other-generations/26844275007/; and Karen Bolser and Rachel Gosciej, "Millennials: Multi-generational Leaders Staying Connected," *Journal of Practical Consulting* 5, no. 2 (Winter 2015): 1–9, https://www.regent.edu/acad/global/publications/jpc/vol5iss2/BolserGosciej.pdf.

14. "Gen Z, Millennials Hit Hardest by Healthcare Costs," Business Wire, October 31, 2019, https://www.businesswire.com/news/home/20191031005089/en/Gen-Z-Millennials-Hit-Hardest-By-Healthcare-Costs.

15. Hillary Hoffower, "Nearly Half of Millennials Have Put Off Needed Medical Care Because They Can't Afford It," *Business Insider*, November 4, 2019, https://www.businessinsider.com/personal-finance/half-of-millennials-delay-medical-care-unaffordable-2019-10.

16. Amy Goyer, "How Years of Caregiving Led to Bankruptcy," AARP, February 26, 2021, https://www.aarp.org/caregiving/financial-legal/info-2021/expenses-financial-strain.html.

17. Flinn, "Millennials: The Emerging Generation."

18. New York Life, "Caregiving and COVID-19."

19. Flinn, "Millennials: The Emerging Generation."

20. "10 Things Millennial Caregivers Should Know About Caring for a Friend or Loved One," SCAN Foundation, https://www.thescanfoundation.org/media/2019/10/giveacare-10things_updated_0926_19.pdf.

21. "Distinctions Between Boomers' and Silent Generation's Financial Security," Stanford Center on Longevity, https://longevity.stanford.edu/wp-content/uploads/2018/06/ch04_Boomers-Silent-Gen-Retirement_JPS-edits_JLS-edit_0620.pdf.

22. Lyle Solomon, "How to Manage Finances as an Unpaid Adult Caregiver," National Council on Aging, April 27, 2023, https://www.ncoa.org/article/how-to-manage-finances-as-an-unpaid-adult-caregiver.

23. "The MetLife Study of Caregiving Costs to Working Caregivers: Double Jeopardy for Baby Boomers Caring for Their Parents," MetLife Mature Market Institute, National Alliance for Caregiving and Center for Long Term Care Research and Policy, New York Medical College, June 2011, https://www.caregiving.org/wp-content/uploads/2011/06/mmi-caregiving-costs-working-caregivers.pdf; and Richard W. Johnson, Karen E. Smith, and Barbara A. Butrica, "Lifetime Employment-Related Costs to Women of Providing Family Care," Urban Institute, February 2023, https://www.dol.gov/sites/dolgov/files/WB/Mothers-Families-Work/Lifetime-caregiving-costs_508.pdf.

24. "Caregiver Statistics: Work and Caregiving," Family Caregiver Alliance, 2016, https://www.caregiver.org/resource/caregiver-statistics-work-and-caregiving/.

25. Simon Workman, "The True Cost of High-Quality Child Care Across the United States," Center for American Progress, June 28, 2021, https://www.americanprogress .org/article/true-cost-high-quality-child-care-across-united-states/.

26. New York Life, "Caregiving and COVID-19."

27. "The Economic Impact of Caregiving," Blue Cross Blue Shield, November 8, 2021, https://www.bcbs.com/the-health-of-america/reports/the-economic-impact-of-care giving#:~:text=The%20estimated%20indirect%20economic%20effect,from%20 absenteeism%20issues%20at%20work; and Dan Witters, "Caregiving Costs U.S. Economy $25.2 Billion in Lost Productivity," Gallup, July 27, 2011, https://news.gallup.com /poll/148670/caregiving-costs-economy-billion-lost-productivity.aspx.

28. Blue Cross Blue Shield, "The Economic Impact of Caregiving."

29. "Medicaid and Home Care: State by State Benefits and Eligibility," Paying for Senior Care, last updated March 8, 2024, https://www.payingforseniorcare.com /medicaid-waivers/home-care.

30. "Introduction to CDPAP Home Care," CDPAPNY, https://cdpapny.org/#intro ductiontocdpap.

Chapter 19: The Changes We Need

1. "Recognize, Assist, Include, Support, & Engage (RAISE) Family Caregivers Act Advisory Council," Administration for Community Living, https://acl.gov /programs/support-caregivers/raise-family-caregiving-advisory-council; and "2022 National Strategy to Support Family Caregivers," RAISE Act Family Caregiving Advisory Council and Advisory Council to Support Grandparents Raising Grandchildren, Administration for Community Living, September 21, 2022, https://acl .gov/sites/default/files/RAISE_SGRG/NatlStrategyToSupportFamilyCaregivers -2.pdf.

2. "Factsheet: What Does the Research Say About Care Infrastructure?" Washington Center for Equitable Growth, April 15, 2021, https://equitablegrowth.org /factsheet-what-does-the-research-say-about-care-infrastructure/.

3. "Fact Sheet: How the Biden-Harris Administration Will Address Our Caregiving Crisis," the White House, https://www.whitehouse.gov/wp-content/uploads/2021/05 /White-House-Caregiving-Fact-Sheet.pdf.

4. Laura Peck, "Policymakers Used to Ignore Child Care. Then Came the Pandemic," *New York Times*, October 6, 2021, https://www.nytimes.com/2021/05/09/business /child-care-infrastructure-biden.html.

5. Elizabeth Bauer, "No, 'Infrastructure of Care' Is Not Infrastructure—and Three Reasons Why It Matters," *Forbes*, April 18, 2021, https://www.forbes.com/sites/ebauer /2021/04/18/no-infrastructure-of-care-is-not-infrastructureand-three-reasons-why -it-matters/.

6. Ai-jen Poo, "Care Has Always Been Infrastructure," *Jezebel*, April 13, 2021, https:// www.jezebel.com/care-has-always-been-infrastructure-1846664603.

7. Anne-Marie Slaughter, "Rosie Could Be a Riveter Only Because of a Care Economy. Where Is Ours?" *New York Times*, April 16, 2021, https://www.nytimes.com/2021/04/16/opinion/care-economy-infrastructure-rosie-the-riveter.html.

8. Becky Little, "The US Funded Universal Childcare During World War II—Then Stopped," History, May 12, 2021, https://www.history.com/news/universal-childcare-world-war-ii.

9. Melinda Gates, "Melinda Gates: This Pandemic Has Exposed Our Nation's Broken Caregiving System," opinion, *Washington Post*, December 2, 2020, https://www.washingtonpost.com/opinions/melinda-gates-broken-caregiving-system/2020/12/02/7c0dd9ae-34d1-11eb-8d38-6aea1adb3839_story.html.

10. The White House, "Caregiving Fact Sheet."

11. Flinn, "Millennials: The Emerging Generation."

Chapter 20: A Bath Bomb Does Not Fix This

1. Roy Remer, "Genuine Resilience Is Closer (and Easier) Than You May Think," webinar, Family Caregiver Alliance, https://www.caregiver.org/resource/genuine-resilience-closer-and-easier-you-may-think-0/.

2. Janneke van Roij et al., "Self-Care, Resilience, and Caregiver Burden."

3. Lourdes Díaz-Rodríguez, Keyla Vargas-Román, Juan Carlos Sanchez-Garcia, Raquel Rodríguez-Blanque, Guillermo Arturo Cañadas-De la Fuente, and Emilia I. De La Fuente-Solana, "Effects of Meditation on Mental Health and Cardiovascular Balance in Caregivers," *International Journal of Environmental Research and Public Health* 18, no. 2 (January 2021): 617, https://doi.org/ 10.3390/ijerph18020617.

4. van Roij et al., "Self-Care, Resilience, and Caregiver Burden."

5. van Roij et al., "Self-Care, Resilience, and Caregiver Burden."

6. "Alzheimer's Disease Caregiver Support Initiative: Evaluation Report Year 1," New York State Department of Health and University at Albany School of Public Health, May 2018, https://www.health.ny.gov/health_care/medicaid/redesign/mrt8004/docs/eval_rpt_y1.pdf.

7. Marie, "Millennials and Mental Health."

8. van Roij et al., "Self-Care, Resilience, and Caregiver Burden."

9. van Roij et al., "Self-Care, Resilience, and Caregiver Burden."

10. "Stress Relief from Laughter? It's No Joke," Stress Management, Mayo Clinic, September 22, 2023, https://www.mayoclinic.org/healthy-lifestyle/stress-management/in-depth/stress-relief/art-20044456.

Chapter 21: How Our *Workplace* Can Help Us (and Themselves)

1. Jeremy Nobel, Jennifer Weiss, Candice Sherman et al., "Supporting Caregivers in the Workplace: A Practical Guide for Employers," AARP and Northeast Business Group on Health (NEBGH) and Solutions Center, September 2022, https://nebgh.org/wp-content/uploads/2017/11/NEBGH-Caregiving_Practical-Guide-FINAL.pdf.

2. Eric Reed, "It's Not Just Tech Companies Anymore, Coke Announces New Family Leave Policy," *TheStreet*, April 11, 2016, https://www.thestreet.com/personal-finance/its-not-just-tech-companies-anymore-coke-announces-new-family-leave-policy-13525842.

3. Joseph B. Fuller and Manjari Raman, "The Caring Company: How Employers Can Cut Costs and Boost Productivity by Helping Employees Manage Caregiving Needs," Harvard Business School, January 16, 2019, https://www.hbs.edu/managing-the -future-of-work/research/Pages/the-caring-company.aspx.

4. AARP and NEBGH, "Supporting Caregivers in the Workplace."

5. AARP and NEBGH, "Supporting Caregivers in the Workplace."

6. AARP and NEBGH, "Supporting Caregivers in the Workplace."

7. Fuller and Raman, "The Caring Company."

8. Fuller and Raman, "The Caring Company."

9. "Something's Gotta Give," Women and the Markets, S&P Global, https://www .spglobal.com/en/research-insights/featured/markets-in-motion/somethings-gotta-give.

10. AARP and NEBGH, "Supporting Caregivers in the Workplace."

11. "What Data Does the BLS Publish on Family Leave?" Employee Benefits, US Bureau of Labor Statistics, updated September 21, 2023, https://www.bls.gov/ebs/fact sheets/family-leave-benefits-fact-sheet.htm.

12. Hamza Shaban and Eli Rosenberg, "Nearly 200 Businesses Urge Congress to Pass Paid Family Leave," *Washington Post*, March 23, 2021, https://www.washingtonpost .com/business/2021/03/23/paid-family-leave-business-leaders/.

13. Molly Weston Williamson, "Self-Employed Workers' Access to State Paid Leave Programs in 2023," Center for American Progress, August 10, 2023, https://www.american progress.org/article/self-employed-workers-access-to-state-paid-leave-programs-in -2023/.

14. Williamson, "Self-Employed Workers' Access."

CHAPTER 22: HOW THE *HEALTHCARE SYSTEM* CAN HELP US

1. Susan C. Reinhard, Heather M. Young, Carol Levine, Kathleen Kelly, Rita Choula, and Jean Accius, "Home Alone Revisited: Family Caregivers Providing Complex Care," AARP Public Policy Institute, April 17, 2019, https://www.aarp.org/ppi/info-2018/home-alone -family-caregivers-providing-complex-chronic-care.html.

2. van Roij et al., "Self-Care, Resilience, and Caregiver Burden."

3. Anne H. Nielsen, Sanne Angel, Ingrid Egerod, "Effect of Relatives' Intensive Care Unit Diaries on Post Traumatic Stress in Patients and Relatives (DRIP-study): A Mixed Methods Study," *Intensive and Critical Care Nursing* 62 (February 2021): 102951, https:// doi.org/10.1016/j.iccn.2020.102951.

4. Hickman and Douglas, "Impact of Chronic Critical Illness."

5. Hickman and Douglas, "Impact of Chronic Critical Illness."

6. Hickman and Douglas, "Impact of Chronic Critical Illness."

7. Anne H. Nielsen, Sanne Angel, Ingrid Egerod, Trine Højfeldt Lund, Marianne Renberg, and Torben Bæk Hansen, "The Effect of Family-Authored Diaries on Posttraumatic Stress Disorder in Intensive Care Unit Patients and Their Relatives: A Randomized Controlled Trial (DRIP-study)," *Australian Critical Care* 33, no. 2 (March 2020): 123–129, https://doi.org/10.1016/j.aucc.2019.01.004; and Nielsen, Angel, and Egerod, "Effect of Relatives' Intensive Care Unit Diaries."

8. Nielsen, Angel, and Egerod, "Effect of Relatives' Intensive Care Unit Diaries."

9. Flinn, "Millennials: The Emerging Generation."

10. Reinhard et al., "Home Alone Revisited."

11. Ashley Stahl, "How Millennials' Views on Healthcare Could Shape the Future of Work," *Forbes*, February 20, 2020, https://www.forbes.com/sites/ashleystahl/2020/02/20 /millennials-views-on-healthcare-and-what-that-means-for-the-future-of-work/.

12. Marion Renault, "'ICU-Delirium' Is Leaving COVID-19 Patients Scared and Confused," *The Atlantic*, May 5, 2020, https://www.theatlantic.com/science/archive /2020/05/coronavirus-icu-delirium/610546/.

Chapter 23: How Systemic Changes Can Facilitate Necessary Care

1. "2022 National Strategy to Support Family Caregivers: Federal Actions," RAISE Act Family Caregiving Advisory Council and Advisory Council to Support Grandparents Raising Grandchildren, September 21, 2022, https://acl.gov/sites/default/files/RAISE _SGRG/NatlStrategyFamCaregivers_FedActions.pdf.

2. RAISE Act Family Caregiving Advisory Council and Advisory Council to Support Grandparents Raising Grandchildren, "2022 National Strategy to Support Family Caregivers."

3. Sarah Stasik and Caring.com, "When to Hire a Geriatric Care Manager for Your Parent," *Next Avenue*, April 6, 2018, https://www.nextavenue.org/hire-geriatric -care-manager-parent/.

4. Stasik and Caring.com, "When to Hire."

5. Stasik and Caring.com, "When to Hire."

6. "Caregiving Consultations & Coaching," CaringKind, https://www.caringkindnyc .org/caregiver-coaching/.

7. Phil Galewitz and Holly K. Hacker, "Medicare's Push to Improve Chronic Care Attracts Business, but Not Many Doctors," NPR, April 17, 2024, https://www.npr.org /sections/health-shots/2024/04/17/1244879040/medicare-chronic-care-management -seniors.

8. "Chronic Care Management Services," mln booklet, Centers for Medicare and Medicaid Services, September 2022, https://www.cms.gov/outreach-and-education /medicare-learning-network-mln/mlnproducts/downloads/chroniccaremanagement .pdf.

9. Galewitz and Hacker, "Medicare's Push to Improve Chronic Care."

10. Galewitz and Hacker, "Medicare's Push to Improve Chronic Care."

11. Alex Olgin and Dan Gorenstein, "Medicare Explores a New Way to Support Caregivers of Dementia Patients," NPR, July 4, 2024, https://www.npr.org/sections/shots -health-news/2024/07/04/nx-s1-5026964/caregivers-dementia-alzheimers-medicare -support.

12. Olgin and Gorenstein, "Medicare Explores a New Way."

13. Olgin and Gorenstein, "Medicare Explores a New Way."

14. Gates, "Melinda Gates: This Pandemic Has Exposed."

INDEX